Unleash Your Mobility

Mastering the Ten Essential Habits for a Life of Freedom and Vitality

By

Rodney M. Casanova

DISCLAIMER

Text copyright© Rodney M. Casanova 2024

Table of Contents

Introduction

In the bustling heart of the city, amidst the symphony of honking cars and hurried footsteps, there exists a hidden sanctuary of movement. Nestled away from the chaos, tucked behind a nondescript storefront, lies a studio pulsating with life. Here, in this haven of motion, individuals from all walks of life converge, drawn by a common desire—to reclaim their mobility and rediscover the freedom that lies within.

Meet Sarah, a vibrant soul with a spirit as boundless as the ocean. Once a fervent dancer, she found herself confined to the confines of a desk job, her body slowly succumbing to the sedentary shackles of modern life. Day after day, she felt the tendrils of stiffness creeping into her muscles, restricting her once-fluid movements and dimming the spark in her eyes.

But deep within Sarah's heart, a flicker of hope remained— a whisper of longing for the days when her body moved with effortless grace and agility. And so, with determined resolve, she embarked on a journey to reignite the flames of her mobility, guided by the wisdom of a book whose title beckoned to her like a beacon in the night—**"Unleash Your Mobility: Mastering Ten Essential Habits for a Life of Freedom and Vitality."**

As Sarah delved into the pages of this transformative tome, she found herself transported into a world where movement was not merely a physical act but a profound expression of vitality and liberation. Each chapter unveiled a new facet of mobility, inviting her to explore the depths of her body's potential and embrace a life of boundless freedom.

From the gentle embrace of daily movement rituals to the exhilarating dance of joint mobility and flexibility, Sarah discovered a treasure trove of practices that revitalized her body and rejuvenated her spirit. With each stretch, each strengthening exercise, she felt the chains of stagnation loosening their grip, replaced by a newfound sense of lightness and fluidity.

But it wasn't just about the physicality of movement; it was about the mindful integration of body, mind, and soul. Through the practice of posture alignment and the cultivation of a strong mind-body connection, Sarah learned to move with intention and purpose, weaving a tapestry of harmony and balance with every step she took.

As the weeks turned into months, Sarah's transformation became a testament to the power of mobility unleashed. No longer bound by the limitations of her sedentary lifestyle, she danced through life with a grace and vitality that seemed to defy gravity itself. Her journey had not only restored her mobility but had ignited a spark within her—a flame of passion and purpose that illuminated the path to a life lived fully and freely.

And Sarah was not alone on this journey. Alongside her stood a community of kindred spirits, each carving their own path to mobility mastery. Together, they celebrated their victories, supported each other through challenges, and bore witness to the profound transformations taking place within and around them.

For in the pages of "Unleash Your Mobility," they had found more than just a book—they had discovered a roadmap to a life of limitless possibilities. With each turn of the page, they unlocked the secrets of their bodies, tapped into the wellsprings of their strength, and embarked on a voyage of self-discovery that would shape their destinies for years to come.

As Sarah closed the book for the final time, a sense of deep gratitude washed over her. Gratitude for the wisdom imparted within its pages, for the journey it had taken her on, and for the newfound freedom that now pulsed through her veins. With a smile gracing her lips and a heart brimming with possibility, she stepped out into the world, ready to dance to the rhythm of her own heartbeat and live a life unleashed.

And so, dear reader, I invite you to join Sarah and countless others on this transformative journey—a journey to unleash your mobility, master the ten essential habits, and embrace a life of freedom and vitality. The adventure awaits. Are you ready to take the first step?

Chapter 1

Setting the Foundation
Recognizing Your Current Mobility Status

In the grand tapestry of life, our bodies are the vessels through which we experience the world—a miraculous amalgamation of muscles, joints, and bones, intricately woven together to facilitate movement and expression. Yet, in the hustle and bustle of modern existence, it's all too easy to overlook the subtle whispers of our bodies, to ignore the signs of imbalance and disconnection that manifest in our movements.

But if we are to embark on a journey of mobility mastery, we must first pause, take stock, and truly listen to what our bodies are trying to tell us. This is where the journey begins—by recognizing our current mobility status and acknowledging the areas in which we may need support and guidance.

The Call of the Body

Imagine waking up one morning to find that your body has become a foreign land—a landscape marked by stiffness, tension, and restricted movement. Perhaps you struggle to bend down and tie your shoes without feeling a twinge in your lower back, or maybe you find it challenging to lift your arms overhead without encountering resistance.

For many of us, these limitations have become an accepted part of our reality—a silent companion that accompanies us through the motions of daily life. But what if we were to heed the call of our bodies, to tune in to the subtle cues and messages they are sending us? What if we were to embark on a journey of self-discovery, guided by the wisdom of our own flesh and blood?

The Mobility Spectrum

Mobility is not a binary state—it exists on a spectrum, ranging from fluidity and ease to stiffness and restriction. At one end of the spectrum lie those blessed with natural grace and agility—the dancers, athletes, and yogis who move with effortless poise and precision. At the other end lie those whose movements are constrained by the accumulated burdens of sedentary living, injury, or illness.

But between these two extremes lies a vast expanse of possibility—a realm where transformation is not only possible but inevitable. It is here, in the liminal space between limitation and liberation, that we find ourselves called to action—to embark on a journey of self-discovery and reclaim the mobility that is our birthright.

The Mobility Assessment

Before we can chart a course toward greater mobility, we must first understand where we currently stand. This is where the mobility assessment comes into play—a tool for gauging our current level of mobility and identifying areas in need of improvement.

The assessment may take various forms, ranging from simple movement tests to more comprehensive evaluations conducted by trained professionals. Regardless of the method used, the goal remains the same—to shine a light on the dark corners of our bodies, to uncover hidden imbalances and restrictions, and to pave the way for targeted interventions and interventions.

Listening to the Body

As we undergo the mobility assessment, it's essential to approach the process with an open mind and a spirit of curiosity. Rather than viewing our limitations as shortcomings, we can reframe them as opportunities for growth and transformation.

Perhaps we discover that our hip flexors are tight from hours spent sitting at a desk, or maybe we find that our shoulders are rounded from years of hunching over a computer screen. Instead of despairing at these revelations, we can celebrate them as milestones on the path to greater awareness and understanding.

Cultivating Mindfulness

Throughout the assessment process, mindfulness emerges as a guiding principle—a reminder to approach our bodies with kindness, compassion, and non-judgment. As we move through the various tests and evaluations, we can cultivate a sense of presence and awareness, tuning in to the subtle nuances of sensation and movement.

In doing so, we become intimate observers of our own experience, learning to read the language of our bodies with greater clarity and precision. With each breath, each movement, we deepen our connection to ourselves, forging a bond that transcends the boundaries of flesh and bone.

Embracing the Journey

As we conclude the mobility assessment, we are left with a clearer understanding of where we stand and where we hope to go. Armed with this knowledge, we can embark on a journey of self-discovery and transformation, guided by the wisdom of our own bodies and the insights gleaned from our assessment.

But this is only the beginning—the first step on a path that stretches far beyond the horizon, beckoning us toward a future filled with possibility and potential. In the chapters that follow, we will explore the essential habits that form the foundation of mobility mastery, each one offering a gateway to greater freedom, vitality, and expression.

So let us set forth on this journey together, with open hearts and willing spirits, ready to embrace the challenges and triumphs that lie ahead. For the road to mobility mastery is not always easy, but it is always worth the journey.

Cultivating the Mindset for Change

In the grand tapestry of human experience, the mind is the architect—the master builder that shapes the contours of our reality and guides the trajectory of our lives. And nowhere is the power of the mind more evident than in the realm of personal transformation. For it is here, in the fertile soil of our thoughts and beliefs, that the seeds of change are sown, taking root and blossoming into the fullness of our potential.

The Power of Mindset

At the heart of any journey of transformation lies the power of mindset—the lens through which we perceive the world and interpret our experiences. In the realm of mobility mastery, cultivating the right mindset is akin to laying a solid foundation for a towering skyscraper—it provides the stability and support necessary to withstand the winds of challenge and adversity.

But what exactly does it mean to cultivate a mindset for change? At its core, it is about adopting a stance of openness, curiosity, and resilience—a willingness to embrace the unknown and venture into uncharted territory. It is about recognizing that change is not only possible but inevitable, and that our thoughts and beliefs play a crucial role in shaping our reality.

The Growth Mindset

Central to the cultivation of a mindset for change is the concept of the growth mindset—a belief in the malleability of our abilities and the potential for growth and improvement. Coined by psychologist Carol Dweck, the growth mindset emphasizes the power of effort, perseverance, and learning from failure in achieving success.

Individuals with a growth mindset view challenges as opportunities for growth, setbacks as temporary obstacles, and feedback as valuable information for improvement. Rather than being discouraged by failure, they see it as a natural part of the learning process—an opportunity to refine their skills and deepen their understanding.

Overcoming Limiting Beliefs

However, cultivating a growth mindset is not without its challenges. For many of us, our minds are riddled with limiting beliefs—deep-seated convictions about our abilities and potential that hold us back from reaching our truest selves. These beliefs often stem from past experiences, societal conditioning, or the influence of others, and can act as barriers to change and growth.

To overcome these limiting beliefs, we must first shine a light on them, bringing them out of the shadows and into the forefront of our awareness. This requires a willingness to engage in honest self-reflection and introspection, to examine the stories we tell ourselves about who we are and what we are capable of achieving.

Once identified, we can begin to challenge these beliefs, questioning their validity and reframing them in a more empowering light. Rather than seeing ourselves as limited by our past experiences or circumstances, we can choose to see them as opportunities for growth and transformation—a springboard from which to launch ourselves into a brighter future.

Embracing the Process

Cultivating a mindset for change is not a one-time event but an ongoing process—a journey of self-discovery and evolution that unfolds over time. It requires patience, persistence, and a willingness to embrace the inherent messiness of growth. It is about showing up each day with an open heart and a curious mind, ready to engage with whatever challenges and opportunities come our way.

In the words of renowned author and motivational speaker Tony Robbins, "It's not what we do once in a while that shapes our lives, but what we do consistently." Indeed, it is through consistent effort and commitment that real change occurs, one small step at a time.

The Power of Visualization

One powerful tool for cultivating a mindset for change is the practice of visualization—a technique used by athletes, performers, and leaders around the world to achieve their goals and unlock their potential. By vividly imagining ourselves succeeding in our endeavors, we can prime our minds for success, building confidence, motivation, and resilience along the way.

Incorporating visualization into our daily routine can help us overcome limiting beliefs, break through mental barriers, and tap into the vast reservoir of untapped potential that lies within us. Whether we are preparing for a challenging workout, a difficult conversation, or a major life transition, visualization can serve as a powerful ally on our journey of transformation.

The Power of Affirmations

Another potent tool for cultivating a mindset for change is the practice of affirmations—positive statements or declarations that we repeat to ourselves to reinforce desired beliefs and behaviors. By affirming our innate worthiness, resilience, and potential, we can reprogram our subconscious minds and align ourselves with the reality we wish to create.

Affirmations can take many forms, from simple statements like "I am capable of achieving my goals" to more specific declarations tailored to our individual needs and desires. By repeating these affirmations regularly, with sincerity and conviction, we can create a powerful feedback loop that strengthens our belief in ourselves and our ability to succeed.

The Role of Community

Finally, cultivating a mindset for change is not something we must do alone. Surrounding ourselves with like-minded individuals who share our vision and support our growth can provide invaluable encouragement, accountability, and inspiration along the way. Whether through online forums, support groups, or in-person communities, connecting with others on a similar journey can help us stay motivated, navigate challenges, and celebrate our successes together.

Creating Your Mobility Blueprint

In the grand tapestry of human experience, the body is our most intimate companion—a vessel through which we navigate the world and express our deepest desires and aspirations. Yet, in the hustle and bustle of modern life, it's all too easy to neglect the needs of our physical selves—to allow the stresses of daily living to chip away at our vitality and rob us of the freedom to move with ease and grace.

But what if we were to reclaim ownership of our bodies—to become architects of our own mobility, crafting a blueprint for a life filled with freedom, vitality, and expression? This is the essence of creating a mobility blueprint—a personalized plan for optimizing our physical well-being and unlocking the full potential of our bodies.

The Importance of a Mobility Blueprint

In the realm of mobility mastery, the creation of a mobility blueprint serves as the cornerstone of our journey—a roadmap that guides us toward greater freedom of movement and expression. It is a living document, continually evolving and adapting to the changing needs and aspirations of our bodies.

But why is a mobility blueprint necessary, you may ask? The answer lies in the complexity of the human body—a miraculous amalgamation of muscles, joints, and connective tissues, each with its unique strengths, weaknesses, and vulnerabilities. By creating a blueprint that takes into account our individual anatomical makeup, movement patterns, and lifestyle factors, we can tailor our approach to mobility enhancement and ensure lasting results.

Assessing Your Mobility Needs

The first step in creating a mobility blueprint is to assess our current level of mobility and identify areas in need of improvement. This requires a willingness to engage in honest self-reflection and introspection—to tune in to the subtle whispers of our bodies and heed the messages they are trying to convey.

There are various methods for assessing mobility, ranging from simple movement tests conducted at home to more comprehensive evaluations performed by trained professionals. Regardless of the method used, the goal remains the same—to gain insight into our strengths and weaknesses, limitations and possibilities, and lay the groundwork for targeted interventions and interventions.

Identifying Mobility Goals

With a clearer understanding of our mobility needs, we can begin to identify our mobility goals—specific outcomes we hope to achieve through our journey of mobility mastery. These goals may vary widely from person to person, ranging from improving flexibility and joint mobility to enhancing strength and stability, or even mastering specific movement skills or activities.

To ensure the effectiveness of our mobility blueprint, it's essential to set goals that are SMART—specific, measurable, attainable, relevant, and time-bound. By articulating our goals in this manner, we can create a clear roadmap for success, track our progress over time, and stay motivated and focused on our journey.

Designing Your Mobility Plan

With our mobility needs and goals in mind, we can now begin to design our mobility plan—a comprehensive strategy for enhancing our physical well-being and unlocking the full potential of our bodies. This plan may encompass various components, including mobility exercises, stretching routines, strength training protocols, and lifestyle modifications, tailored to our individual needs and preferences.

When designing our mobility plan, it's essential to take a holistic approach, addressing not only the physical aspects of mobility but also the mental, emotional, and spiritual dimensions of our well-being. By nurturing all aspects of our being, we can create a foundation for lasting health and vitality and ensure that our mobility journey is both fulfilling and sustainable.

Incorporating Mobility Practices

With our mobility plan in hand, the next step is to begin incorporating mobility practices into our daily routine. This may involve setting aside dedicated time each day for mobility exercises and stretching routines, integrating movement breaks into our workday, or finding creative ways to incorporate mobility-enhancing activities into our daily lives.

It's essential to approach our mobility practices with an open mind and a spirit of curiosity, exploring different modalities and techniques to find what works best for us. Whether it's yoga, Pilates, tai chi, or functional movement training, there are countless paths to mobility mastery, and it's up to us to find the ones that resonate most deeply with our bodies and souls.

Cultivating Consistency and Persistence

As we embark on our journey of mobility mastery, it's essential to cultivate consistency and persistence in our practice. Like tending to a garden, our bodies require regular care and attention to flourish and thrive. By committing to our mobility practices day in and day out, we can gradually chip away at our limitations, expand our range of motion, and unlock new levels of freedom and expression.

But consistency alone is not enough—we must also cultivate persistence in the face of challenges and setbacks. There will inevitably be days when we feel tired, unmotivated, or discouraged by our progress. In those moments, it's essential to remind ourselves of our overarching vision and purpose, to draw strength from the knowledge that every step we take brings us closer to our goals

Seeking Support and Guidance

Finally, creating a mobility blueprint is not something we must do alone. There are countless resources available to support us on our journey, from books and online courses to mobility coaches and physical therapists. By seeking out support and guidance from those who have walked the path before us, we can accelerate our progress, avoid common pitfalls, and stay motivated and inspired along the way.

Chapter 2

Habit 1 - Daily Movement Rituals
The Power of Consistent Movement

In the grand tapestry of life, movement is the thread that weaves together the fabric of our existence—a symphony of motion that shapes our experiences, fuels our passions, and connects us to the world around us. Yet, in the frenetic pace of modern living, it's all too easy to become disconnected from our bodies—to neglect the fundamental need for daily movement and allow the sedentary shackles of modernity to encroach upon our vitality.

But what if we were to reclaim movement as a sacred ritual—a daily practice that nourishes our bodies, enlivens our spirits, and aligns us with the rhythm of life itself? This is the essence of Habit 1—Daily Movement Rituals—a foundational practice that forms the cornerstone of our journey toward mobility mastery.

The Power of Consistent Movement

At the heart of Habit 1 lies the power of consistent movement—a commitment to incorporating physical activity into our daily lives, regardless of the circumstances or challenges we may face. Consistent movement is not merely a means to an end but a way of being—a fundamental aspect of our humanity that shapes our physical, mental, and emotional well-being.

But what exactly constitutes consistent movement, you may ask? It's not about running marathons or lifting heavy weights (though those activities certainly have their place), but rather about finding ways to move our bodies in ways that feel good and nourishing to us. It could be as simple as taking a brisk walk in nature, practicing yoga or tai chi, dancing to our favorite music, or playing with our children or pets.

The Benefits of Consistent Movement

The benefits of consistent movement are myriad, extending far beyond the physical realm to encompass every aspect of our being. From improved cardiovascular health and enhanced flexibility to reduced stress and anxiety, the rewards of daily movement are as diverse as they are profound.

Physiologically, consistent movement helps to lubricate our joints, strengthen our muscles, and improve our posture and balance. It boosts our immune system, increases our energy levels, and promotes better sleep. Mentally and emotionally, it releases endorphins—the body's natural feel-good chemicals—and fosters a sense of well-being, confidence, and resilience.

But perhaps most importantly, consistent movement reconnects us to the wisdom of our bodies—to the innate intelligence that guides us toward health and vitality. It reminds us that we are not merely observers of life but active participants, co-creators of our own destinies.

Overcoming Barriers to Consistent Movement

Despite the myriad benefits of consistent movement, many of us struggle to incorporate it into our daily lives. We may be hindered by time constraints, lack of motivation, or physical limitations, or we may simply be unaware of the profound impact that daily movement can have on our well-being.

To overcome these barriers, it's essential to approach consistent movement with a spirit of curiosity, creativity, and adaptability. Rather than viewing it as a chore or obligation, we can reframe it as an opportunity for self-care and self-expression—a sacred ritual that honors the inherent wisdom of our bodies.

One way to overcome barriers to consistent movement is to integrate it into our daily routines in small, manageable increments. This could mean taking short movement breaks throughout the day, scheduling regular walks or workouts into our calendars, or finding ways to incorporate movement into our daily activities, such as standing while talking on the phone or taking the stairs instead of the elevator.

Cultivating Mindful Movement

Another key aspect of consistent movement is cultivating mindfulness—the practice of being fully present and aware of our bodies and surroundings as we move. Mindful movement invites us to tune in to the sensations of our bodies, to notice the subtle nuances of movement, and to savor the experience of being alive.

To cultivate mindfulness in our movement practice, we can start by paying attention to our breath—the rhythmic flow of inhalation and exhalation that serves as our anchor in the present moment. As we move, we can synchronize our breath with our movements, allowing it to guide and inform our actions.

We can also bring awareness to the sensations of our bodies as we move—noticing the feeling of our feet connecting with the ground, the stretch of our muscles as we reach and extend, and the rhythm of our heartbeat as it quickens with exertion. By bringing mindful awareness to our movement practice, we can deepen our connection to ourselves and cultivate a sense of presence and vitality that extends far beyond the mat or gym.

Designing Your Personal Movement Routine

In the bustling tapestry of modern life, where schedules are packed and demands are relentless, the concept of carving out time for movement may seem like a luxury reserved for the few. Yet, amidst the chaos and clamor, lies a profound truth—movement is not a luxury but a necessity, an essential component of our physical, mental, and emotional well-being.

In Chapter 2 of our journey toward mobility mastery, we delve into the heart of Habit 1—Daily Movement Rituals. Here, we explore the art and science of designing a personal movement routine—a sacred practice that nourishes our bodies, enlivens our spirits, and aligns us with the rhythm of life itself.

The Importance of Daily Movement Rituals

At the core of Habit 1 lies the recognition that movement is not something to be relegated to the sidelines of our lives but woven into the very fabric of our existence. Daily movement rituals provide us with an opportunity to reconnect with our bodies, to honor the innate wisdom that resides within us, and to cultivate a deeper sense of presence and vitality.

But why are daily movement rituals important, you may ask? The answer lies in the transformative power of consistency—a commitment to showing up for ourselves each day, regardless of the obstacles or distractions that may arise. By making movement a non-negotiable part of our daily routine, we lay the foundation for lasting health and vitality, and unlock the full potential of our bodies.

Designing Your Personal Movement Routine

The beauty of daily movement rituals lies in their flexibility and adaptability. There is no one-size-fits-all approach to movement, no cookie-cutter routine that works for everyone. Instead, we are invited to become architects of our own mobility, crafting a personalized movement routine that honors the unique needs and desires of our bodies.

To design your personal movement routine, it's essential to start by clarifying your goals and intentions. What do you hope to achieve through your daily movement practice? Are you looking to improve flexibility, build strength, reduce stress, or simply reconnect with your body? By articulating your goals clearly, you can tailor your routine to align with your aspirations and aspirations.

Assessing Your Mobility Needs

Next, take some time to assess your current level of mobility and identify areas in need of improvement. This could involve performing simple movement tests to gauge your flexibility, strength, and balance, or seeking feedback from a qualified movement professional.

As you assess your mobility needs, pay attention to any areas of tension, stiffness, or discomfort that may arise. These are valuable clues that can help guide your movement practice and inform the selection of exercises and techniques that will best serve your body.

Exploring Different Modalities

Once you have clarified your goals and assessed your mobility needs, it's time to explore different modalities and techniques that resonate with you. There are countless ways to move our bodies, each offering its unique blend of benefits and challenges.

For example, you may choose to incorporate yoga into your routine for its focus on flexibility, balance, and mindfulness. Or perhaps you're drawn to strength training for its ability to build lean muscle mass and improve overall body composition. Other options include Pilates, dance, martial arts, tai chi, qigong, and more.

Creating a Balanced Routine

As you explore different modalities, aim to create a balanced routine that addresses all aspects of fitness—flexibility, strength, cardiovascular endurance, and balance. This could involve incorporating a mix of resistance training, cardiovascular exercise, and mobility work into your routine, with an emphasis on variety and progression.

For example, you might start your routine with a dynamic warm-up to mobilize your joints and activate your muscles, followed by a combination of strength training exercises targeting major muscle groups. You could then finish with a cool-down consisting of stretching and relaxation techniques to promote recovery and reduce muscle soreness.

Listening to Your Body

Throughout the design process, it's essential to listen to your body and honor its feedback. Pay attention to how different movements feel in your body—whether they create sensations of ease and openness or tension and discomfort. Use this information to adjust your routine as needed, modifying exercises, and techniques to better suit your body's unique needs.

Remember that progress is not always linear, and there will be days when you feel stronger and more flexible than others. Be gentle with yourself and avoid pushing through pain or discomfort. Instead, focus on cultivating a sense of presence and mindfulness in your movement practice, tuning in to the subtle cues and messages that your body is sending you.

Incorporating Mindfulness and Intention

Finally, infuse your movement routine with mindfulness and intention, approaching each session as a sacred ritual and an opportunity for self-discovery and growth. Begin by setting an intention for your practice—a guiding principle or affirmation that aligns with your goals and aspirations.

Throughout your routine, cultivate a sense of presence and awareness, focusing your attention on the sensations of your body as you move. Notice the feeling of your feet connecting with the ground, the stretch of your muscles as you reach and extend, and the rhythm of your breath as it flows in and out of your body.

Integrating Movement into Daily Life

In the cacophony of modern existence, where the demands of work, family, and obligations often vie for our attention, the notion of finding time for dedicated exercise can seem like an elusive dream. Yet, amidst the chaos and busyness of life, lies a simple truth—movement is not something to be confined to the confines of a gym or fitness class but can be seamlessly integrated into the fabric of our daily lives.

In Chapter 2 of our journey toward mobility mastery, we delve into the heart of Habit 1—Daily Movement, exploring the art and science of integrating movement into our daily routines. Here, we discover that movement is not merely a means to an end but a way of being—a sacred practice that nourishes our bodies, enlivens our spirits, and infuses every moment with vitality and joy.

The Myth of Exercise as Separate from Daily Life

For many of us, the concept of exercise has become synonymous with structured workouts performed in designated spaces at specific times of the day. We carve out time from our busy schedules to visit the gym, attend a fitness class, or go for a run, viewing exercise as a separate activity distinct from the rest of our lives.

But what if we were to challenge this paradigm—to reframe exercise not as a separate entity but as an integral part of our daily lives? This is the essence of Habit 1—Daily Movement—an invitation to infuse every moment with the joy of movement, to find opportunities for activity in the most mundane of tasks, and to reclaim our bodies as vehicles for expression and exploration.

The Power of Micro-Movements

At the heart of integrating movement into daily life lies the recognition that even the smallest of movements can have a profound impact on our well-being. Whether it's taking the stairs instead of the elevator, parking further away from our destination, or incorporating short movement breaks into our workday, micro-movements offer a simple yet powerful way to increase physical activity levels and promote overall health.

Research has shown that even brief periods of activity throughout the day can help to reduce the risk of chronic diseases such as heart disease, diabetes, and obesity, as well as improve mood, concentration, and productivity. By embracing the power of micro-movements, we can transform the most mundane of tasks into opportunities for growth and transformation, and infuse our daily lives with vitality and joy.

Creating Movement Friendly Environments

In addition to rethinking our daily routines, creating movement-friendly environments can also play a crucial role in integrating movement into daily life. This could involve making simple changes to our physical surroundings, such as setting up a standing desk at work, investing in ergonomic furniture, or designing our living spaces to encourage movement and activity.

For example, rather than sitting on the couch to watch TV, we can opt for a more active seating option, such as a stability ball or a cushion on the floor. We can also create designated areas in our homes for movement and exercise, such as a yoga mat in the living room or a set of resistance bands in the bedroom, making it easy to incorporate physical activity into our daily routine.

Embracing Active Transportation

Another powerful way to integrate movement into daily life is by embracing active forms of transportation, such as walking, cycling, or using public transit. Not only does active transportation offer a sustainable and environmentally friendly alternative to driving, but it also provides an opportunity to increase physical activity levels and improve overall health and well-being.

For example, rather than driving to work or running errands, we can opt to walk or bike whenever possible, enjoying the fresh air, sunshine, and scenery along the way. We can also use public transit as an opportunity to incorporate movement into our daily routine, such as taking the stairs instead of the escalator or walking to the bus stop or train station.

Incorporating Movement into Social Activities

Finally, integrating movement into daily life can also be a social endeavor, offering an opportunity to connect with others while engaging in physical activity. Whether it's going for a hike with friends, playing a game of soccer with colleagues, or taking a dance class with a partner, movement-based social activities provide a fun and enjoyable way to stay active and connected.

By incorporating movement into our social activities, we not only reap the physical benefits of exercise but also enjoy the social and emotional rewards of spending time with others. Whether it's sharing a laugh, supporting each other through challenges, or celebrating our achievements together, movement-based social activities offer a powerful way to nourish our bodies, minds, and spirits.

Chapter 3

Habit 2 - Mindful Stretching Practices
The Art of Stretching for Mobility

In the grand tapestry of movement mastery, stretching is the thread that weaves together the fabric of flexibility, mobility, and vitality. It is a practice that transcends the physical realm, inviting us to journey inward, explore the depths of our bodies, and unlock the untapped potential that resides within us. In Chapter 3 of our quest for mobility mastery, we delve into the heart of Habit 2—Mindful Stretching Practices—the art of stretching for mobility.

The Essence of Mindful Stretching

At its core, mindful stretching is more than just a physical practice—it is a holistic approach to mobility that engages the body, mind, and spirit in a dance of exploration and self-discovery. It is a practice that invites us to cultivate presence, awareness, and compassion as we move through a series of stretches, honoring the innate wisdom of our bodies and embracing the journey of transformation that unfolds with each breath.

But what exactly does it mean to practice mindful stretching? At its essence, mindful stretching is about tuning in to the sensations of our bodies as we move, noticing the subtle nuances of tension and release, and responding with kindness and curiosity to whatever arises. It is about approaching our practice with an open heart and a beginner's mind, ready to explore the vast landscape of our inner world and discover the limitless potential that resides within us.

The Benefits of Mindful Stretching

The benefits of mindful stretching are myriad, extending far beyond the physical realm to encompass every aspect of our being. Physically, mindful stretching helps to improve flexibility, mobility, and range of motion, reducing the risk of injury and enhancing performance in other physical activities. It also helps to alleviate muscle tension, improve posture, and promote relaxation, making it an invaluable tool for managing stress and anxiety.

Mentally and emotionally, mindful stretching offers a sanctuary for self-care and self-reflection, providing a sacred space for us to connect with ourselves and nurture our inner landscape. It invites us to cultivate mindfulness, presence, and self-compassion as we move through our practice, fostering a sense of inner peace and well-being that extends far beyond the mat.

The Principles of Mindful Stretching

At the heart of mindful stretching lie a set of guiding principles that inform our practice and shape our experience. These principles serve as signposts along the journey of mobility mastery, offering wisdom and guidance as we navigate the terrain of our inner world and explore the depths of our bodies.

1. **Presence: Mindful stretching begins with presence—** the act of bringing our awareness fully into the present moment, tuning in to the sensations of our bodies as we move. By cultivating presence in our practice, we create a foundation for self-discovery and transformation, allowing us to connect more deeply with ourselves and the world around us.

2. **Breath**: Breath is the life force that animates our bodies and fuels our practice of mindful stretching. By syncing our breath with our movements, we harness the power of the breath to guide and inform our practice, facilitating relaxation, expansion, and release. Breath becomes our anchor in the present moment, guiding us back to ourselves whenever our minds wander or our bodies resist.

3.**Awareness**: Awareness is the cornerstone of mindful stretching—the ability to observe our thoughts, feelings, and sensations without judgment or attachment. By cultivating awareness in our practice, we gain insight into the patterns and habits that shape our experience, allowing us to respond with kindness and curiosity to whatever arises.

4. **Intention:** Intention is the driving force behind our practice of mindful stretching—the guiding principle or aspiration that informs our movements and shapes our experience. By setting an intention for our practice, we create a framework for growth and transformation, aligning our actions with our deepest values and aspirations.

5. **Compassion**: Compassion is the heart of mindful stretching—the practice of extending kindness and understanding to ourselves and others as we move through our practice. By cultivating compassion in our practice, we create a safe and nurturing space for exploration and self-discovery, allowing us to embrace our imperfections and celebrate our progress with grace and humility.

The Art of Stretching for Mobility

Now that we've explored the principles of mindful stretching, let's dive into the art of stretching for mobility—the practice of using stretching techniques to enhance flexibility, mobility, and range of motion in the body. While there are countless stretching techniques and modalities to choose from, here are some key principles to keep in mind as you explore the world of stretching for mobility:

1. **Dynamic vs. Static Stretching**: Dynamic stretching involves moving the body through a range of motion in a controlled and deliberate manner, while static stretching involves holding a stretch for a period of time without movement. Both dynamic and static stretching have their place in a comprehensive stretching routine, with dynamic stretching serving as a warm-up for physical activity and static stretching serving as a cool-down for relaxation and recovery.

2. **Active vs. Passive Stretching**: Active stretching involves using the muscles themselves to move the body into a stretch, while passive stretching involves using external forces, such as gravity or props, to facilitate the stretch. Both active and passive stretching can be effective for improving flexibility and mobility, and it's important to explore both approaches to find what works best for your body.

3. **Proprioceptive Neuromuscular Facilitation (PNF):** PNF stretching is a technique that involves a combination of stretching and contracting the muscles to facilitate relaxation

and release. It can be performed with a partner or on your own and is particularly effective for improving flexibility and range of motion in specific muscle groups.

4. **Breath Awareness**: Breath awareness is a key component of stretching for mobility, helping to facilitate relaxation, expansion, and release in the body. By syncing your breath with your movements, you can create a sense of flow and ease in your practice, allowing you to move more deeply into the stretch and explore new levels of flexibility and mobility.

5. **Mindfulness and Presence:** Finally, mindfulness and presence are essential elements of tretching for mobility, helping to cultivate a sense of awareness and connection as you move through your practice. By tuning in to the sensations of your body and observing your thoughts and feelings without judgment, you can create a safe and nurturing space for exploration and self-discovery, allowing you to unlock the full potential of your body and embrace the journey of mobility mastery.

Integrating Mindful Stretching into Daily Life

Now that we've explored the principles and techniques of mindful stretching, let's explore how we can integrate this practice into our daily lives, weaving it into the fabric of our existence and infusing every moment with presence, awareness, and vitality.

1. **Morning Rituals:** Start your day with a gentle stretching routine to awaken your body and mind, preparing yourself for the day ahead. Focus on dynamic movements that promote circulation and mobility, such as sun salutations, cat-cow stretches, and spinal twists.

2. **Movement Breaks:** Take regular movement breaks throughout the day to counteract the effects of sitting and sedentary behavior. Incorporate simple stretches and mobility exercises into your routine, such as shoulder rolls, neck stretches, and hip openers, to keep your body feeling loose and limber.

3. **Active Commuting:** Use your daily commute as an opportunity to incorporate movement into your routine. Walk or bike to work whenever possible, or take the stairs instead of the elevator to

sneak in some extra activity throughout the day.

4. **Mindful Movement Practices**: Explore mindful movement practices such as yoga, tai chi, or qigong, which combine stretching, breath awareness, and meditation to cultivate presence, balance, and inner peace. These practices

offer a holistic approach to mobility that nourishes the body, mind, and spirit.

5. **Evening Rituals**: Wind down your day with a soothing stretching routine to release tension and prepare your body for restorative sleep. Focus on passive stretches and relaxation techniques, such as gentle forward folds, hip openers, and deep breathing exercises, to promote relaxation and recovery.

Understanding Different Stretching Techniques

Stretching is not just about reaching for your toes or trying to touch your nose to your knees. It's a multifaceted practice that encompasses various techniques, each offering its own benefits and serving different purposes. In Chapter 3, we delve into the world of mindful stretching practices, exploring the diverse array of techniques available to enhance flexibility, mobility, and overall well-being.

The Importance of Understanding Stretching Techniques

Before delving into the specifics of different stretching techniques, it's essential to understand why stretching matters. Stretching is not just about improving flexibility or preparing for physical activity; it's about cultivating a deeper connection with our bodies, enhancing body awareness, and promoting overall health and well-being.

By understanding different stretching techniques, we can tailor our stretching routine to meet our individual needs, address specific areas of tension or tightness, and maximize the benefits of our practice. Whether you're a seasoned yogi or a beginner to stretching, there's something for everyone to discover in the world of mindful stretching practices.

Dynamic Stretching

Dynamic stretching involves moving the body through a range of motion in a controlled and deliberate manner, using momentum and muscle activation to increase flexibility and mobility. Unlike static stretching, which involves holding a stretch for a prolonged period, dynamic stretching is more dynamic and fluid, making it an excellent choice for warming up the body before physical activity.

One of the key benefits of dynamic stretching is that it helps to increase blood flow and circulation to the muscles, warming them up and preparing them for movement. It also helps to improve joint mobility and range of motion, making it easier to perform activities that require flexibility and agility.

Some common examples of dynamic stretching exercises include leg swings, arm circles, lunges with a twist, and high knees. These exercises can be performed individually or as part of a dynamic stretching routine, and can be adapted to suit your fitness level and goals.

Static Stretching

Static stretching involves holding a stretch for a prolonged period, typically 15-30 seconds, without movement. It is often used to improve flexibility, increase range of motion, and alleviate muscle tension and tightness. Unlike dynamic stretching, which focuses on moving the body through a range of motion, static stretching targets specific muscle groups and aims to lengthen and relax the muscles.

One of the key benefits of static stretching is that it allows for deep relaxation and release in the muscles, helping to reduce muscle tension and improve overall flexibility. It also helps to improve joint mobility and range of motion, making it easier to perform everyday activities and prevent injury.

Some common examples of static stretching exercises include hamstring stretches, quadriceps stretches, calf stretches, and shoulder stretches. These exercises can be performed individually or as part of a comprehensive stretching routine, and should be held for a minimum of 15-30 seconds to allow for adequate muscle relaxation and lengthening.

Proprioceptive Neuromuscular Facilitation (PNF)

Proprioceptive Neuromuscular Facilitation (PNF) is a stretching technique that involves a combination of stretching and contracting the muscles to facilitate relaxation and release. It is often used to improve flexibility, increase range of motion, and alleviate muscle tightness and tension. PNF stretching can be performed with a partner or on your own and is particularly effective for targeting specific muscle groups and enhancing overall mobility.

One of the key benefits of PNF stretching is that it helps to improve muscle coordination and proprioception, the body's ability to sense its position in space. By alternating between stretching and contracting the muscles, PNF stretching helps to enhance the brain's awareness of muscle length and tension, making it easier to relax and release tight muscles.

Some common examples of PNF stretching techniques include contract-relax, hold-relax, and contract-relax-agonist-contract (CRAC). These techniques involve a combination of passive stretching, active contraction, and relaxation, and should be performed with caution to avoid overstretching or injury.

Ballistic Stretching

Ballistic stretching involves using momentum and bouncing movements to increase flexibility and range of motion. It is often used by athletes and dancers to improve performance and enhance agility and coordination. Unlike static stretching, which involves holding a stretch for a prolonged period, ballistic stretching is more dynamic and explosive, making it an excellent choice for athletes who require quick and powerful movements.

One of the key benefits of ballistic stretching is that it helps to improve muscle elasticity and responsiveness, allowing for greater range of motion and flexibility. It also helps to increase blood flow and circulation to the muscles, warming them up and preparing them for intense physical activity.

Some common examples of ballistic stretching exercises include leg swings, arm swings, and torso twists. These exercises should be performed with caution, as they can increase the risk of injury if done incorrectly or excessively. It's essential to start slowly and gradually increase the intensity and range of motion to avoid straining the muscles or joints.

Active Isolated Stretching (AIS)

Active Isolated Stretching (AIS) is a stretching technique that involves actively contracting the muscles opposite the ones being stretched. It is often used to improve flexibility, increase range of motion, and alleviate muscle tightness and tension. AIS targets specific muscle groups and aims to lengthen and relax the muscles gradually, allowing for deeper and more effective stretching.

One of the key benefits of AIS is that it helps to improve muscle coordination and proprioception, making it easier to control and stabilize the body during movement. It also helps to increase blood flow and circulation to the muscles, promoting relaxation and release.

Some common examples of AIS exercises include hamstring stretches, quadriceps stretches, calf stretches, and shoulder stretches. These exercises should be performed with caution to avoid overstretching or injury, and it's essential to listen to your body and stop if you experience any pain or discomfort.

Yin Yoga

Yin Yoga is a slow-paced style of yoga that involves holding passive stretches for an extended period, typically 3-5 minutes or longer. It is often used to improve flexibility, increase joint mobility, and promote relaxation and stress relief. Yin Yoga targets the connective tissues of the body, such as ligaments, tendons, and fascia, and aims to release tension and tightness in these tissues gradually.

One of the key benefits of Yin Yoga is that it helps to improve flexibility and range of motion in the joints, making it easier to perform everyday activities and prevent injury. It also helps to increase circulation and blood flow to the connective tissues, promoting healing and recovery.

Some common examples of Yin Yoga poses include seated forward fold, pigeon pose, sphinx pose, and butterfly pose. These poses should be held for an extended period to allow for deep relaxation and release in the connective tissues, and it's essential to listen to your body and avoid pushing yourself beyond your limits.

Choosing the Right Stretching Technique

With so many stretching techniques to choose from, it can be challenging to know which one is right for you. The key is to listen to your body and choose techniques that feel good and suit your individual needs and goals. Whether you're looking to improve flexibility, increase range of motion, or alleviate muscle tension and tightness, there's a stretching technique out there for you.

When selecting a stretching technique, consider factors such as your fitness level, flexibility, and any pre-existing injuries or conditions. Start slowly and gradually increase the intensity and duration of your stretches, and always listen to your body and stop if you experience any pain or discomfort.

Implementing Stretching into Your Daily Routine

Stretching is not just a physical practice; it's a gateway to greater flexibility, mobility, and overall well-being. In Chapter 3, we delve into the practical aspects of mindful stretching practices, exploring how to integrate stretching into your daily routine seamlessly. From morning rituals to bedtime stretches, we'll uncover the myriad ways to weave stretching into the fabric of your daily life, ensuring that you reap the full benefits of this transformative practice.

Understanding the Importance of Daily Stretching

Before we delve into the specifics of implementing stretching into your daily routine, it's essential to understand why daily stretching matters. Daily stretching offers a multitude of benefits for both the body and mind, including:

1. **Improved Flexibility**: Daily stretching helps to increase flexibility by lengthening and relaxing the muscles, making it easier to perform everyday activities and preventing injury.

2. **Enhanced Mobility**: Stretching improves joint mobility and range of motion, allowing for greater ease of movement and reducing the risk of stiffness and pain.

3. **Stress Relief**: Stretching promotes relaxation and stress relief by releasing tension in the muscles and calming the nervous system, helping to alleviate the physical and mental effects of stress.

4. **Improved Posture: Stretching helps to correct imbalances in the muscles and improve posture by lengthening tight muscles and strengthening weak muscles, promoting better alignment and reducing the risk of injury.

5.Increased Energy Levels: Stretching increases blood flow and circulation to the muscles, delivering oxygen and nutrients and promoting a sense of vitality and well-being.

Morning Stretching Rituals

Starting your day with a gentle stretching routine is a powerful way to awaken your body and mind, preparing yourself for the day ahead. Incorporating stretching into your morning routine can help to increase energy levels, improve focus and concentration, and set a positive tone for the day.

Here are some tips for implementing morning stretching into your daily routine:

1. **Set Aside Time**: Set aside 10-15 minutes each morning for a stretching routine. This could be before or after your morning shower, or even while you're still in bed.

2. **Start Slow**: Begin with gentle stretches that target major muscle groups, such as the hamstrings, quadriceps, calves, and shoulders. Move slowly and mindfully, paying attention to the sensations in your body as you stretch.

3. **Focus on Breath**: Use your breath to guide your movements, inhaling deeply as you lengthen and exhaling fully as you release. This helps to oxygenate the muscles and promote relaxation.

4. **Listen to Your Body**: Pay attention to how your body feels as you stretch, and adjust the intensity of your stretches accordingly. Avoid pushing yourself too hard or forcing your body into uncomfortable positions.

5. **Combine with Mindfulness**: Incorporate mindfulness techniques into your stretching routine, such as body scanning or mindful breathing, to cultivate presence and awareness.

Stretching Breaks Throughout the Day

In addition to incorporating stretching into your morning routine, it's essential to take regular stretching breaks throughout the day to counteract the effects of sitting and sedentary behavior. Sitting for long periods can lead to tightness and stiffness in the muscles, which can contribute to poor posture, decreased mobility, and increased risk of injury.

Here are some tips for incorporating stretching breaks into your daily routine:

1. **Set Reminders**: Set reminders on your phone or computer to take stretching breaks every hour or so. This could be a simple alarm or a notification that pops up on your screen.

2. **Desk Stretches**: Perform simple stretches at your desk to relieve tension and tightness in the muscles. This could include neck stretches, shoulder rolls, chest openers, and seated spinal twists.

3. **Take Movement Breaks**: Instead of sitting for long periods, take short movement breaks to stretch and move your body. This could involve walking around the office, doing a few yoga poses, or taking a quick dance break.

4. **Use Props**: Keep stretching props such as resistance bands or yoga blocks at your desk to help facilitate deeper stretches and increase range of motion.

5. **Incorporate Mindfulness**: Use stretching breaks as an opportunity to practice mindfulness and relaxation techniques, such as deep breathing or progressive muscle relaxation.

Evening Stretching Rituals

Just as morning stretching prepares you for the day ahead, evening stretching helps to unwind and relax your body, preparing you for restorative sleep. Incorporating stretching into your evening routine can help to release tension and tightness accumulated throughout the day, promote relaxation, and improve sleep quality.

Here are some tips for implementing evening stretching into your daily routine:

1. **Set Aside Time:** Set aside 10-15 minutes each evening for a stretching routine. This could be before or after dinner, or as part of your bedtime routine.

2. **Focus on Relaxation**: Choose gentle stretches that promote relaxation and release, such as forward folds, gentle twists, and hip openers. Avoid intense or vigorous stretches that may interfere with your ability to unwind and relax.

3. **Combine with Mindfulness**: Use stretching as an opportunity to practice mindfulness and relaxation techniques, such as deep breathing or body scanning. Focus on the sensations in your body as you stretch, and let go of any tension or tightness you may be holding onto.

4. **Promote Sleep**: Choose stretches that promote relaxation and prepare your body for sleep, such as gentle backbends, seated forward folds, and supine twists. Hold each stretch for a minimum of 30 seconds to allow for deep relaxation and release.

5. **Create a Ritual**: Create a ritual around your evening stretching routine to signal to your body that it's time to unwind and relax. This could involve dimming the lights,

playing soft music, or lighting a candle to create a calming atmosphere.

Weekend Stretching Sessions

In addition to incorporating stretching into your daily routine, it's also beneficial to set aside time for longer stretching sessions on the weekends. Weekend stretching sessions allow you to focus on deeper stretches, target specific areas of tension or tightness, and explore new stretching techniques and modalities.

Here are some tips for incorporating weekend stretching sessions into your routine:

1. **Schedule Time:** Schedule a longer stretching session on the weekend when you have more time to dedicate to your practice. This could be a Saturday morning or Sunday evening, depending on your schedule and preferences.

2. **Set Intentions:**Set intentions for your weekend stretching session, such as improving flexibility, releasing tension, or exploring new stretching techniques. This helps to focus your practice and guide your movements.

3. **Explore New Techniques**: Use weekend stretching sessions as an opportunity to explore new stretching techniques and modalities. Try out different styles of yoga,

experiment with PNF stretching, or incorporate props such as foam rollers or massage balls into your routine.

4. **Listen to Your Body**: Pay attention to how your body feels as you stretch and adjust your practice accordingly. If you experience any pain or discomfort, back off from the stretch or modify it to suit your needs.

5. **Combine with Self-Care**: Use weekend stretching sessions as a form of self-care and relaxation. Combine stretching with other self-care practices such as meditation, aromatherapy, or a warm bath to create a nurturing and rejuvenating experience.

Chapter 4

Habit 3 - Strengthening Your Foundation Building Strength for Stability

In the grand symphony of movement mastery, strength forms the sturdy backbone upon which the body's intricate dance unfolds. In Chapter 4, we delve into the essence of building strength for stability, exploring the foundational principles and practical strategies for cultivating a resilient and stable body. From core stability to functional strength, we'll uncover the keys to fortifying your foundation and unlocking the full potential of your body.

Understanding the Importance of Strength for Stability

Before we embark on our journey of building strength for stability, it's essential to understand why strength matters. Strength is more than just the ability to lift heavy weights or perform impressive feats—it's the foundation upon which all movement is built. Without strength, our bodies lack the stability and support needed to perform everyday activities and prevent injury.

Strength training plays a crucial role in maintaining muscle mass, bone density, and overall health as we age. It helps to improve posture, balance, and coordination, reducing the risk of falls and injuries. It also enhances athletic performance, allowing athletes to perform at their best and achieve their goals.

Core Stability: The Key to a Strong Foundation

At the heart of strength for stability lies core stability—the ability to maintain a stable and neutral spine during movement. The core muscles, including the abdominals, obliques, and lower back muscles, act as a stabilizing force, providing support and stability to the spine and pelvis during dynamic movements.

Core stability is essential for maintaining proper alignment and posture, reducing the risk of back pain and injury, and enhancing athletic performance. It also serves as the foundation for all other movements, providing a stable base from which to generate power and force.

Practical Strategies for Building Core Stability

Building core stability requires a combination of strength training, balance exercises, and functional movements. Here are some practical strategies for strengthening your core and improving stability:

1. **Planks**: Planks are one of the most effective exercises for building core stability. Start by holding a plank position for 30 seconds to 1 minute, gradually increasing the duration as you build strength.

2. **Russian Twists**: Russian twists target the obliques and help to improve rotational stability. Sit on the floor with your knees bent and feet flat on the ground, lean back slightly, and twist your torso from side to side while holding a weight or medicine ball.

3. **Dead Bugs**: Dead bugs are a great exercise for improving core stability and coordination. Lie on your back with your arms extended overhead and legs lifted in tabletop position, lower one arm and the opposite leg towards the ground, then return to the starting position and repeat on the other side.

4. **Bird Dogs**: Bird dogs target the core muscles and help to improve stability and balance. Start on your hands and knees, extend one arm and the opposite leg, then return to the starting position and repeat on the other side.

5. **Pilates**: Pilates is a great way to improve core stability and overall strength. Incorporate Pilates exercises such as the hundred, roll-ups, and leg circles into your routine to target the core muscles and enhance stability.

Functional Strength: The Key to Everyday Movement

In addition to core stability, building functional strength is essential for everyday movement and activities. Functional strength refers to the ability to perform activities of daily living with ease and efficiency, such as lifting, bending, squatting, and reaching.

Functional strength training focuses on compound movements that mimic real-life activities, such as squats, lunges, deadlifts, and rows. These exercises engage multiple muscle groups simultaneously, helping to improve strength, stability, and coordination.

Practical Strategies for Building Functional Strength

Here are some practical strategies for building functional strength and enhancing everyday movement:

1. **Squats:** Squats are one of the best exercises for building lower body strength and functional movement patterns. Start with bodyweight squats, then progress to goblet squats, front squats, and back squats as you build strength.

2. **Lunges**: Lunges target the lower body and help to improve balance, stability, and coordination. Start with stationary lunges, then progress to walking lunges, reverse lunges, and lateral lunges as you build strength.

3. **Deadlifts**: Deadlifts are a great exercise for building posterior chain strength and functional movement patterns. Start with kettlebell deadlifts or Romanian deadlifts, then progress to barbell deadlifts as you build strength and confidence.

4. **Rows:** Rows target the upper back and help to improve posture, stability, and shoulder health. Start with bodyweight rows or dumbbell rows, then progress to barbell rows or cable rows as you build strength.

5. **Push-Ups**: Push-ups are a compound exercise that targets the chest, shoulders, and triceps, as well as the core muscles for stability. Start with modified push-ups on your knees or against a wall, then progress to full push-ups as you build strength.

Integrating Strength Training into Your Daily Routine

Now that we've explored the importance of strength for stability and practical strategies for building core stability and functional strength, let's discuss how to integrate strength training into your daily routine.

1. **Set Goals**: Set specific, measurable goals for your strength training routine, such as increasing the number of push-ups you can perform or lifting a certain amount of weight. Having clear goals will help to keep you motivated and focused on your progress.

2. **Create a Schedule**: Schedule your strength training workouts into your weekly routine, just like you would any other appointment or commitment. This will help to ensure that you make time for your workouts and stay consistent with your training.

3. **Mix It Up**: Incorporate a variety of exercises and modalities into your strength training routine to keep things interesting and prevent boredom. This could include bodyweight exercises, free weights, resistance bands, or machine-based exercises.

4. **Listen to Your Body**: Pay attention to how your body feels during and after your workouts, and adjust your routine

accordingly. If you're feeling fatigued or sore, take a rest day or focus on lighter, lower-intensity exercises.

. 5. **Stay Consistent:** Consistency is key when it comes to strength training. Aim to work out at least 3-4 times per week, and gradually increase the intensity and duration of your workouts as you build strength and confidence.

Targeted Exercises for Mobility

In the dynamic tapestry of movement, mobility acts as the brushstroke that paints the canvas of our physical experience. It's the freedom to move effortlessly, the grace to navigate life's twists and turns with ease. In Chapter 4, we dive into the essence of strengthening your foundation through targeted exercises for mobility. From joint mobility to functional movements, we uncover the keys to unlocking the full range of motion and embracing the fluidity of the human body.

Understanding the Importance of Mobility

Before delving into the specifics of targeted exercises for mobility, it's crucial to understand why mobility matters. Mobility is more than just the ability to touch your toes or perform a split—it's the foundation of all movement. Without adequate mobility, our bodies become stiff, rigid, and prone to injury.

Mobility encompasses flexibility, stability, and strength, working together harmoniously to create fluid and efficient movement patterns. It allows us to perform everyday tasks with ease, whether it's bending down to tie our shoes, reaching for a high shelf, or playing sports with friends.

Joint Mobility: The Key to Fluid Movement

At the heart of mobility lies joint mobility—the ability of our joints to move freely and smoothly through their full range of motion. Joint mobility is essential for maintaining healthy joints, preventing stiffness and pain, and optimizing movement efficiency.

Each joint in the body has its own unique range of motion and movement patterns, determined by its anatomical structure and surrounding muscles and ligaments. By improving joint mobility, we can enhance overall movement quality, reduce the risk of injury, and improve performance in physical activities.

Practical Strategies for Improving Joint Mobility

Improving joint mobility requires a combination of targeted exercises, dynamic movements, and mindful awareness. Here are some practical strategies for improving joint mobility:

1. **Joint Circles**: Perform joint circles to lubricate the joints and improve mobility. Start with small circles and gradually increase the size and range of motion as you warm up.

2. **Dynamic Stretching**: Incorporate dynamic stretching exercises into your warm-up routine to improve joint mobility and flexibility. This could include leg swings, arm circles, and torso twists.

3. **Foam Rolling**: Use a foam roller to release tension and tightness in the muscles and fascia, improving joint mobility and flexibility. Focus on areas of tension or tightness, such as the calves, hamstrings, and hips.

4. **Mobility Drills**: Perform mobility drills that target specific joints and movement patterns, such as shoulder dislocates, hip circles, and ankle mobilizations. These drills help to improve joint mobility and range of motion.

5. **Yoga and Pilates**:Practice yoga and Pilates to improve joint mobility, flexibility, and stability. These mind-body practices incorporate dynamic movements, stretching, and breathwork to enhance overall movement quality and promote relaxation and stress relief.

Functional Movements: The Key to Everyday Mobility

In addition to joint mobility, functional movements play a crucial role in improving everyday mobility. Functional movements are movements that mimic real-life activities and require multiple muscle groups to work together synergistically.

By incorporating functional movements into our daily routine, we can improve movement efficiency, reduce the risk of injury, and enhance overall mobility and quality of life.

Practical Strategies for Incorporating Functional Movements

Here are some practical strategies for incorporating functional movements into your daily routine:

1. **Squat Variations**: Perform squat variations such as bodyweight squats, goblet squats, and pistol squats to improve lower body strength, mobility, and stability. Focus

on maintaining proper form and alignment throughout the movement.

2. **Lunge Variations:** Incorporate lunge variations such as forward lunges, reverse lunges, and lateral lunges to improve lower body strength, balance, and coordination. Experiment with different foot positions and ranges of motion to target different muscle groups.

3. **Hinge Variations**: Practice hinge variations such as Romanian deadlifts, kettlebell swings, and single-leg deadlifts to improve hip mobility, hamstring flexibility, and posterior chain strength. Focus on hinging at the hips while maintaining a neutral spine and engaged core.

4. **Push and Pull Movements**: Include push and pull movements such as push-ups, rows, and pull-ups to improve upper body strength, mobility, and stability. Focus on engaging the chest, back, and shoulder muscles while maintaining proper form and alignment.

5.**Carrying and Crawling**: Incorporate carrying and crawling exercises such as farmer's walks, bear crawls, and crab walks to improve core stability, shoulder mobility, and coordination. Experiment with different loads and distances to challenge your body in new ways.

Integrating Targeted Mobility Exercises into Your Daily Routine

Now that we've explored the importance of mobility and practical strategies for improving joint mobility and functional movements, let's discuss how to integrate targeted mobility exercises into your daily routine.

1. **Set Aside Time**:Set aside dedicated time each day to perform targeted mobility exercises. This could be in the morning as part of your morning routine, during your lunch break, or in the evening before bed.

2. **Start Slow**: Begin with gentle mobility exercises and gradually increase the intensity and duration as you warm up. Focus on quality over quantity, and listen to your body to avoid overexertion or injury.

3. **Focus on Problem Areas**: Pay attention to areas of tension or tightness in your body and prioritize mobility exercises that target those areas. This could include tight hips, shoulders, or ankles, which are common problem areas for many people.

4. **Combine with Other Activities**:

Incorporate mobility exercises into other activities throughout your day, such as stretching while watching TV, foam rolling after a workout, or practicing yoga during your lunch break.

5. **Stay Consistent**: Consistency is key when it comes to improving mobility. Aim to perform targeted mobility exercises regularly, ideally daily or several times per week, to see the best results.

Incorporating Strength Training into Your Lifestyle

Strength training is not just about building muscles; it's about cultivating resilience, fortifying your foundation, and embracing the full potential of your body. In Chapter 4, we delve into the essence of incorporating strength training into your lifestyle. From setting goals to finding motivation, we uncover the keys to making strength training a sustainable and fulfilling part of your everyday life.

Understanding the Power of Strength Training

Strength training is a cornerstone of physical fitness, offering a multitude of benefits for both body and mind. Beyond building muscle mass and strength, strength training enhances bone density, improves metabolic health, and boosts mood and cognitive function.

Strength training also plays a crucial role in injury prevention and rehabilitation, helping to correct muscular imbalances, improve joint stability, and reduce the risk of falls and injuries. Additionally, strength training enhances athletic performance, allowing athletes to perform at their peak and achieve their goals.

Setting Goals: The Foundation of Success

Before embarking on your strength training journey, it's essential to set clear and achievable goals. Goals provide direction and motivation, helping to keep you focused and on track with your training.

When setting goals for strength training, consider factors such as:

Specificity: Clearly define what you want to achieve with your strength training, whether it's building muscle, improving strength, or enhancing athletic performance.

Measurability Set measurable benchmarks to track your progress and assess your success. This could include increasing the amount of weight lifted, improving the number of repetitions performed, or reducing body fat percentage.

Attainability: Ensure that your goals are realistic and attainable, given your current fitness level, lifestyle, and resources. Break larger goals down into smaller, manageable steps to make them more achievable.

Relevance: Align your strength training goals with your overall health and fitness objectives, as well as your personal interests and preferences. Choose goals that resonate with you and inspire you to take action.

Finding Motivation: Cultivating the Fire Within

Maintaining motivation is essential for staying committed to your strength training routine. While motivation may ebb and flow over time, there are several strategies you can use to keep the fire burning:

1. **Set Meaningful Goals**: Choose goals that are personally meaningful and align with your values and aspirations. Visualize the benefits of achieving your goals and use them as fuel to keep you motivated.

2. **Celebrate Progress**: Celebrate your progress along the way, no matter how small. Recognize and acknowledge your achievements, whether it's reaching a new personal best, completing a challenging workout, or sticking to your training schedule.

3. **Find Accountability:** Accountability can be a powerful motivator in sticking to your strength training routine. Partnering with a workout buddy, joining a group fitness class, or hiring a personal trainer can help to keep you accountable and motivated.

4. **Mix It Up**: Keep your strength training routine fresh and exciting by incorporating variety into your workouts. Try new exercises, change up your training split, or explore different training modalities to keep things interesting and prevent boredom.

5. **Stay Consistent:** Consistency is key when it comes to building strength and seeing results. Commit to showing up for your workouts regularly, even on days when you don't feel like it, and trust in the process.

Designing Your Strength Training Program

Once you've set your goals and found your motivation, it's time to design your strength training program. A well-designed program should be tailored to your individual needs, goals, and preferences, and should include a variety of exercises to target all major muscle groups.

Here are some key components to consider when designing your strength training program:

1. **Exercise Selection**: Choose a variety of compound and isolation exercises to target different muscle groups and movement patterns. Compound exercises, such as squats, deadlifts, and bench presses, engage multiple muscle groups simultaneously and are great for building overall strength and muscle mass. Isolation exercises, such as bicep curls, tricep extensions, and calf raises, target specific muscle groups and are useful for addressing weak points or imbalances.

2. **Training Frequency**: Determine how often you'll be training each muscle group per week. Aim for at least 2-3 days of strength training per week, with a day or two of rest in between workouts to allow for recovery. Splitting your workouts into upper body and lower body days, or focusing on different muscle groups on different days, can help to optimize recovery and maximize results.

3. **Intensity:** Choose an appropriate intensity for each exercise, based on your individual strength level and training goals. For strength and muscle building, aim to work at a moderate to high intensity, lifting heavy enough weights to fatigue the muscles within 8-12 repetitions. For muscular endurance and toning, aim for higher repetitions with lighter weights.

4. **Volume:** Determine the number of sets and repetitions you'll perform for each exercise, as well as the rest intervals between sets. Aim for 2-4 sets of each exercise, with 8-12 repetitions per set for muscle building, and 12-20 repetitions per set for muscular endurance. Rest for 1-2 minutes between sets to allow for adequate recovery.

5. **Progression:** Gradually increase the intensity and volume of your workouts over time to continue challenging your muscles and stimulating growth. This could involve increasing the weight lifted, performing more repetitions, or decreasing rest intervals between sets.s

Integrating Strength Training into Your Lifestyle

Now that you've designed your strength training program, it's time to integrate it into your lifestyle. Here are some tips for making strength training a sustainable and enjoyable part of your everyday life:

1. **Schedule Your Workouts:** Treat your strength training workouts like any other appointment or commitment and schedule them into your calendar. Choose times that work best for you, whether it's first thing in the morning,

during your lunch break, or in the evening after work.

2. **Prepare in Advance**: Lay out your workout clothes, pack your gym bag, and prepare any equipment or accessories you'll need for your workouts in advance. Having everything ready to go will make it easier to get started and stay on track with your training.

3. **Create a Workout Space**:Set up a dedicated workout space at home or find a gym that you enjoy training at. Make sure your workout space is clean, organized, and free from distractions, allowing you to focus fully on your training.

4. **Find a Workout Partner**: Partnering with a friend, family member, or coworker can make strength training more fun and enjoyable. Having someone to train with can provide motivation, accountability, and support, making it easier to stick to your workouts and achieve your goals.

5. **Stay Flexible**: Be flexible with your strength training routine and be willing to adapt and adjust as needed. Life can be unpredictable, and there may be times when you need to modify your workouts or skip a session altogether. Instead of getting discouraged, focus on staying consistent over the long term and making progress at your own pace.

Chapter 5

Habit 4 - Joint Mobility and Flexibility Enhancing Joint Health for Greater Mobility

In the intricate tapestry of movement, our joints serve as the hinges that allow us to bend, twist, and flex with fluidity and grace. In Chapter 5, we embark on a journey into the realm of joint mobility and flexibility, exploring the profound impact of healthy joints on our overall mobility and well-being. From understanding the anatomy of our joints to practical strategies for enhancing joint health, we uncover the keys to unlocking greater mobility and freedom of movement.

Understanding the Anatomy of Joints

Before delving into the specifics of enhancing joint health, it's essential to understand the anatomy of our joints. Joints are the points in the body where two or more bones meet, allowing for movement and flexibility. There are several types of joints in the body, each with its own unique structure and function:

1. **Synovial Joints**: Synovial joints are the most common type of joint in the body and are characterized by a fluid-filled cavity called the synovial cavity. Examples of synovial joints include the shoulder, hip, knee, and elbow joints.

2. **Cartilaginous Joints**: Cartilaginous: joints are connected by cartilage and allow for slight movement. Examples of cartilaginous joints include the intervertebral discs of the spine and the pubic symphysis.

3. **Fibrous Joints**: Fibrous joints are connected by fibrous tissue and allow for minimal to no movement. Examples of fibrous joints include the sutures of the skull and the joints between the teeth and the jawbone.

The Importance of Joint Health

Healthy joints are essential for maintaining mobility, stability, and overall quality of life. When our joints are healthy and functioning optimally, we can move with ease and perform everyday activities without pain or restriction. However, when our joints become stiff, inflamed, or damaged, it can lead to pain, discomfort, and decreased mobility.

Enhancing joint health is essential for preventing injury, reducing the risk of degenerative conditions such as osteoarthritis, and promoting overall well-being. By incorporating targeted exercises, lifestyle modifications, and mindful practices into our daily routine, we can optimize joint health and unlock the full potential of our bodies.

Practical Strategies for Enhancing Joint Health

Improving joint health requires a multifaceted approach that addresses both physical and lifestyle factors. Here are some practical strategies for enhancing joint health:

1. **Stay Active**: Regular physical activity is essential for maintaining healthy joints and preventing stiffness and immobility. Engage in a variety of low-impact activities such

as walking, swimming, cycling, and yoga to promote joint mobility and flexibility.

2. **Strengthen Muscles Around Joints**: Strengthening the muscles surrounding your joints helps to provide support and stability, reducing the risk of injury and improving joint function. Focus on exercises that target the muscles around specific joints, such as leg lifts for the hips and squats for the knees.

3. **Maintain a Healthy Weight**: Excess weight puts added stress on the joints, increasing the risk of joint pain, inflammation, and degenerative conditions such as osteoarthritis. Maintain a healthy weight through a balanced diet and regular exercise to reduce strain on the joints and improve overall joint health.

4. **Practice Good Posture**: Poor posture can lead to misalignment of the joints and increased stress on the muscles and ligaments surrounding them. Practice good posture by standing tall, keeping your shoulders back and relaxed, and engaging your core muscles to support your spine.

5. **Stay Hydrated**: Adequate hydration is essential for maintaining healthy joints, as water helps to lubricate the joints and cushion the bones during movement. Drink plenty

of water throughout the day to keep your joints hydrated and functioning optimally.

Joint Mobility Exercises

Incorporating joint mobility exercises into your daily routine is an effective way to improve joint health and flexibility. These exercises help to increase range of motion, reduce stiffness, and promote fluid movement of the joints. Here are some examples of joint mobility exercises for various parts of the body:

1. **Shoulder Circles**: Stand tall with your arms relaxed at your sides. Slowly circle your shoulders forward, then backward, making large, smooth circles with your shoulders. Repeat for 10-15 repetitions.

2. **Hip Circles**: Stand with your feet hip-width apart and hands on your hips. Circle your hips clockwise, then counterclockwise, making large, smooth circles with your hips. Repeat for 10-15 repetitions.

3. **Ankle Circles**: Sit on the floor with your legs extended in front of you. Circle your ankles clockwise, then counterclockwise, making large, smooth circles with your ankles. Repeat for 10-15 repetitions.

4. **Wrist Flexion and Extension**: Extend your arms in front of you with your palms facing down. Slowly bend your wrists upward, then downward, feeling a gentle stretch in your wrists and forearms. Repeat for 10-15 repetitions.

5. **Neck Rotations**: Sit tall with your shoulders relaxed. Slowly turn your head to the right, then to the left, keeping your chin parallel to the ground. Repeat for 10-15 repetitions on each side.

Flexibility Exercises

In addition to joint mobility exercises, incorporating flexibility exercises into your routine can further enhance joint health and range of motion. Flexibility exercises help to lengthen the muscles and improve overall flexibility, reducing the risk of injury and promoting optimal joint function. Here are some examples of flexibility exercises:

1. **Hamstring Stretch**: Sit on the floor with one leg extended in front of you and the other leg bent, foot resting against the inner thigh of the extended leg. Lean forward from the hips, reaching towards your toes. Hold for 30 seconds, then switch sides.

2. **Quadriceps Stretch**: Stand tall with your feet hip-width apart. Bend one knee and bring your heel towards your glutes, grasping your ankle with your hand. Gently pull your heel towards your glutes until you feel a stretch in the front of your thigh. Hold for 30 seconds, then switch sides.

3.**Chest Stretch**: Stand tall with your feet hip-width apart and interlace your fingers behind your back. Straighten your arms and lift them away from your body, feeling a stretch in your chest and shoulders. Hold for 30 seconds.

4. **Calf Stretch**: Stand facing a wall with one foot in front of the other. Place your hands on the wall at shoulder height and lean forward, keeping your back leg straight and heel on the ground. Feel a stretch in your calf muscle. Hold for 30 seconds, then switch sides.

5. **Spinal Twist**: Sit tall on the floor with your legs extended in front of you. Bend your right knee and place your right foot

on the outside of your left knee. Twist your torso to the right, placing your left elbow on the outside of your right knee and looking over your right shoulder. Hold for 30 seconds, then switch sides.

Lifestyle Modifications for Joint Health

In addition to exercise, making lifestyle modifications can further support joint health and mobility. Here are some lifestyle tips for promoting healthy joints:

1. **Eat a Balanced Diet**: A balanced diet rich in fruits, vegetables, lean proteins, and healthy fats provides essential nutrients for joint health, such as omega-3 fatty acids, vitamin D, and antioxidants.

2. **Manage Stress**: Chronic stress can contribute to muscle tension and joint stiffness. Practice stress-reducing techniques such as deep breathing, meditation, yoga, and spending time in nature to promote relaxation and reduce stress levels.

3. **Get Adequate Sleep**: Sleep is essential for tissue repair and regeneration, including the muscles and joints. Aim for 7-9 hours of quality sleep per night to support joint health and overall well-being.

4. **Avoid Overuse and Injury**: Be mindful of overuse injuries and avoid activities that place excessive strain on the joints, such as repetitive movements, heavy lifting, and high-impact exercises. Listen to your body and give yourself time to rest and recover when needed.

5. **Stay Active Throughout the Day**: Incorporate movement into your daily routine to keep your joints lubricated and flexible. Take short breaks to stretch and move around throughout the day, whether it's walking, standing, or doing gentle exercises.

Techniques for Improving Joint Flexibility

In the intricate dance of movement, joint flexibility is the graceful choreography that allows us to bend, twist, and stretch with ease and fluidity. In Chapter 5, we embark on a journey into the realm of joint mobility and flexibility, exploring the profound impact of supple joints on our overall well-being. From understanding the mechanics of joint flexibility to practical techniques for enhancing range of motion, we uncover the keys to unlocking greater freedom and fluidity in our movements.

Understanding Joint Flexibility

Before delving into techniques for improving joint flexibility, it's essential to understand what flexibility is and why it matters. Flexibility refers to the ability of a joint to move through its full range of motion without restriction or discomfort. It is influenced by factors such as muscle length, joint structure, and connective tissue elasticity.

Joint flexibility plays a crucial role in maintaining optimal movement patterns, reducing the risk of injury, and enhancing athletic performance. When our joints are flexible, we can move with greater ease and efficiency, whether it's reaching for a high shelf, bending down to tie our shoes, or performing dynamic movements in sports and exercise.

Factors Affecting Joint Flexibility

Several factors can affect joint flexibility, including:

1. **Muscle Length**: The length of the muscles surrounding a joint plays a significant role in joint flexibility. Tight or shortened muscles can restrict joint movement and limit flexibility, while lengthened muscles allow for greater range of motion.

2. **Joint Structure**: The structure of a joint, including its shape, size, and alignment, can influence its flexibility. Some joints naturally have a greater range of motion than others due to their anatomical structure.

3. **Connective Tissue Elasticity**: Connective tissues such as ligaments, tendons, and fascia play a crucial role in joint flexibility. Healthy connective tissues are elastic and allow for smooth movement of the joints, while stiff or tight

connective tissues can restrict movement and limit flexibility.

4. **Age:** As we age, joint flexibility tends to decrease due to changes in muscle elasticity, joint lubrication, and connective tissue quality. However, regular stretching and mobility exercises can help to maintain and improve flexibility as we age.

Techniques for Improving Joint Flexibility

Improving joint flexibility requires a combination of stretching, mobility exercises, and lifestyle modifications. Here are some practical techniques for enhancing joint flexibility:

1. **Static Stretching**: Static stretching involves holding a stretch in a stationary position for a prolonged period, typically 15-30 seconds. This type of stretching helps to lengthen the muscles and improve joint flexibility. Examples of static stretches include hamstring stretches, quadriceps stretches, and shoulder stretches.

2. **Dynamic Stretching**: Dynamic stretching involves moving a joint through its full range of motion in a controlled manner, typically in a repetitive fashion. This type of stretching helps to improve joint mobility and prepare the

body for movement. Examples of dynamic stretches include leg swings, arm circles, and torso twists.

3. **Proprioceptive Neuromuscular Facilitation (PNF):** PNF stretching techniques involve a combination of stretching and contracting the muscles to improve flexibility. This type of stretching is often done with a partner and can be highly effective for improving joint flexibility. Examples of PNF stretching techniques include contract-relax and hold-relax stretches.

4. **Foam Rolling:** Foam rolling involves using a foam roller to apply pressure to tight or restricted areas of the body, releasing tension and improving joint mobility. Foam rolling can be particularly beneficial for enhancing flexibility in areas such as the hips, thighs, and calves.

5. **Yoga and Pilates:** Yoga and Pilates are mind-body practices that incorporate stretching, strength, and mobility exercises to improve flexibility and overall well-being. Both disciplines emphasize breath awareness, proper alignment, and mindful movement, making them effective tools for enhancing joint flexibility.

6. **Active Isolated Stretching (AIS):** AIS is a stretching technique that involves actively contracting the muscles opposite the ones being stretched to facilitate greater flexibility. This technique helps to lengthen the muscles and improve joint mobility without causing strain or discomfort.

Lifestyle Modifications for Improved Flexibility

In addition to stretching exercises, making lifestyle modifications can further enhance joint flexibility. Here are some lifestyle tips for promoting greater flexibility:

1. **Stay Hydrated**: Adequate hydration is essential for maintaining healthy joints and connective tissues. Drink plenty of water throughout the day to keep your joints lubricated and flexible.

2. **Eat a Balanced Diet**: A balanced diet rich in nutrients such as vitamins, minerals, and antioxidants supports joint health and overall

well-being. Include plenty of fruits, vegetables, whole grains, and lean proteins in your diet to nourish your joints and muscles.

3. **Manage Stress**: Chronic stress can contribute to muscle tension and stiffness, affecting joint flexibility. Practice stress-reducing techniques such as deep breathing, meditation, and yoga to promote relaxation and reduce tension in the muscles and joints.

4. **Get Adequate Sleep**: Quality sleep is essential for tissue repair and recovery, including the muscles and joints. Aim for 7-9 hours of sleep per night to support joint health and optimize recovery from exercise and physical activity.

5. **Stay Active**: Regular physical activity helps to maintain joint mobility and flexibility by keeping the muscles and connective tissues supple and healthy. Incorporate a variety of activities into your routine, including stretching, strength training, and cardiovascular exercise, to promote overall flexibility and well-being.

Joint Mobility Drills for Daily Practice

In the intricate tapestry of movement, joint mobility is the vital thread that allows us to bend, twist, and rotate with grace and ease. In Chapter 5, we delve into the realm of joint mobility and flexibility, exploring the profound impact of daily mobility drills on our overall well-being. From understanding the importance of joint mobility to practical drills for enhancing flexibility, we uncover the keys to unlocking greater freedom and fluidity in our movements.

The Importance of Joint Mobility

Before delving into joint mobility drills, it's essential to understand why joint mobility matters. Joint mobility refers to the ability of a joint to move freely and smoothly through its full range of motion. It is influenced by factors such as muscle length, joint structure, and connective tissue elasticity.

Maintaining optimal joint mobility is essential for several reasons:

1.**Preventing Injury**: Improved joint mobility reduces the risk of injury by allowing for smoother, more efficient movement patterns. When our joints move freely, we are less likely to experience strain, sprains, or other musculoskeletal injuries.

2. **Enhancing Performance:** Optimal joint mobility enhances athletic performance by improving agility, coordination, and range of motion. Athletes with greater joint mobility can move more efficiently and effectively, leading to better overall performance in sports and physical activities.

3. **Reducing Pain and Discomfort**: Stiff or restricted joints can lead to pain, discomfort, and decreased quality of life. By improving joint mobility, we can alleviate tension, reduce stiffness, and promote overall comfort and well-being.

4. **Supporting Joint Health**: Regular joint mobility drills help to maintain the health and integrity of our joints. By moving our joints through their full range of motion on a regular basis, we promote synovial fluid circulation, improve joint lubrication, and nourish the surrounding tissues.

Chapter 6

Habit 5 - Balancing Mobility and Stability
Finding the Equilibrium Between Mobility and Stability

In the intricate interplay of movement, the balance between mobility and stability is the cornerstone of optimal function and performance. In Chapter 6, we embark on a journey to explore the delicate equilibrium between these two essential components of movement. From understanding the roles of mobility and stability to practical strategies for finding balance, we uncover the keys to unlocking greater strength, flexibility, and resilience in our bodies.

The Yin and Yang of Movement

Understanding Mobility and Stability

Before delving into the nuances of balancing mobility and stability, it's essential to understand the fundamental principles of each:

1. **Mobility**: Mobility refers to the ability of a joint to move freely and smoothly through its full range of motion. It is influenced by factors such as muscle length, joint structure, and connective tissue elasticity. Optimal mobility allows for fluid movement patterns and dynamic flexibility, essential for activities such as running, dancing, and yoga.

2. **Stability:** Stability, on the other hand, refers to the ability of a joint to remain stable and supported during movement. It is provided by the surrounding muscles, ligaments, and tendons, which work together to stabilize the joint and prevent excessive movement or instability. Optimal stability is crucial for maintaining proper alignment, preventing injury, and supporting functional movement patterns.

The Importance of Balancing Mobility and Stability

Finding the right balance between mobility and stability is essential for several reasons:

1. **Injury Prevention:** Imbalances between mobility and stability can increase the risk of injury by compromising joint integrity and movement efficiency. For example, excessive mobility without sufficient stability can lead to joint instability and increased susceptibility to sprains, strains, and other musculoskeletal injuries.

2. **Performance Enhancement**: Balancing mobility and stability enhances athletic performance by optimizing movement mechanics, coordination, and power generation. Athletes with balanced mobility and stability can move with greater efficiency, power, and precision, leading to improved performance in sports and physical activities.

3. **Functional Movement:** In everyday life, we rely on a combination of mobility and stability to perform a wide range of activities, from walking and lifting to reaching and bending. Balancing mobility and stability allows us to move with ease and confidence, whether we're navigating obstacles, carrying groceries, or playing with our children.

Practical Strategies for Balancing Mobility and Stability

Achieving a harmonious balance between mobility and stability requires a multifaceted approach that addresses both physical and neuromuscular factors. Here are some practical strategies for finding equilibrium:

1. **Assessment and Awareness**: Start by assessing your current level of mobility and stability in various joints and movement patterns. Pay attention to areas of imbalance or restriction and identify any compensatory patterns or weaknesses that may be contributing to imbalances.

2. **Mobility Exercises**: Incorporate targeted mobility exercises into your routine to improve joint mobility and flexibility. Focus on areas of tightness or restriction, such as the hips, shoulders, and spine, and perform dynamic stretches, foam rolling, and joint mobilizations to release tension and improve range of motion.

3. **Stability Training**: Implement stability training exercises to strengthen the muscles surrounding the joints and improve joint stability. Include exercises that target the core, hips, shoulders, and ankles, such as planks, bridges, lunges, and rotator cuff exercises, to build strength, control, and proprioception.

4. Functional Movement Patterns

Practice functional movement patterns that integrate mobility and stability, such as squats, lunges, hinges, and rotations. Focus on maintaining proper alignment, control, and stability throughout each movement, and progress gradually as you build strength and confidence.

5.Balance and Proprioception

Incorporate balance and proprioception exercises into your routine to enhance joint awareness and stability. Include exercises such as single-leg balance, stability ball exercises, and balance board drills to challenge your balance and improve neuromuscular control.

Integrating Mobility and Stability into Daily Life

Finding balance between mobility and stability is not just about performing specific exercises—it's about integrating these principles into our daily lives and movement practices. Here are some practical tips for incorporating mobility and stability into your daily routine:

1. **Mindful Movement:** Practice mindful movement throughout the day by paying attention to your posture, alignment, and movement patterns. Take breaks to stretch, move, and reset your posture regularly, especially if you spend long periods sitting or standing.

2. **Functional Training**: Emphasize functional training exercises that mimic real-life movement patterns and activities. Choose exercises that require a combination of mobility and stability, such as squatting, bending, lifting, and reaching, to reinforce balanced movement patterns and support functional performance.

3. **Variety and Adaptation**: Incorporate a variety of movement modalities and exercises into your routine to challenge your body in different ways and prevent

stagnation. Adapt your workouts to suit your individual needs and goals, and listen to your body to avoid overtraining or injury.

4. Recovery and Regeneration

Prioritize recovery and regeneration practices such as rest, hydration, nutrition, and self-care to support optimal mobility and stability. Allow your body time to rest and recover between workouts, and prioritize activities that promote relaxation and stress relief.

5. **Consistency and Patience**: Be consistent in your mobility and stability training efforts, but also be patient and realistic in your expectations. Building balanced mobility and stability takes time, dedication, and consistent effort, so stay committed to your practice and trust in the process.

Exercises for Improving Balance and Coordination

In the intricate dance of movement, balance and coordination are the silent orchestrators that guide our every step, jump, and twist. In Chapter 6, we delve into the realm of balancing mobility and stability by exploring exercises that enhance balance and coordination. From understanding the importance of balance and coordination to practical drills for improving these skills, we uncover the keys to unlocking greater strength, agility, and resilience in our bodies.

The Significance of Balance and Coordination

Before delving into the exercises, let's understand why balance and coordination are crucial components of movement:

1. **Balance**: Balance refers to the ability to maintain equilibrium and stability while stationary or in motion. It involves the coordination of sensory information from the vestibular system, proprioceptive system, and visual system to make precise adjustments and maintain postural control. Optimal balance is essential for preventing falls, supporting functional movement patterns, and enhancing athletic performance.

2. **Coordination**: Coordination refers to the ability to synchronize muscle actions and movements to achieve a specific task or goal. It involves the integration of sensory information, motor control, and cognitive processes to execute movements with precision and fluidity. Optimal coordination is essential for performing complex movements, such as running, jumping, and throwing, with efficiency and accuracy.

The Role of Balance and Coordination in Daily Life

Balance and coordination play a crucial role in various activities of daily living, sports, and physical activities:

1. **Everyday Activities**: Maintaining balance and coordination is essential for performing everyday activities such as walking, standing, bending, and reaching. Whether navigating stairs, carrying groceries, or getting out of bed, we rely on balanced movement patterns to move safely and efficiently through our environment.

2. **Sports and Recreation**: In sports and recreational activities, balance and coordination are fundamental for optimal performance. Athletes rely on precise balance and coordination to execute movements such as dribbling a basketball, swinging a golf club, or performing gymnastics routines with speed, power, and control.

3. **Injury Prevention**: Improving balance and coordination can help reduce the risk of injury by enhancing neuromuscular control, proprioception, and postural stability. By training the body to respond effectively to

changes in position, terrain, and external stimuli, we can minimize the likelihood of falls, slips, and other accidents.

Practical Exercises for Improving Balance and Coordination

Now that we understand the importance of balance and coordination, let's explore some practical exercises for improving these skills:

1. Single-Leg Balance:

- Stand tall with your feet hip-width apart.

- Shift your weight onto one leg and lift the opposite foot off the ground, balancing on the standing leg.

- Find a focal point to gaze at to help maintain balance.

- Hold the position for 30-60 seconds, then switch sides.

- To progress, try closing your eyes or adding arm movements while balancing.

2. **Balance Pad Exercises**:

- Stand on a balance pad or foam cushion with your feet hip-width apart.

- Maintain your balance as you perform various movements, such as squats, lunges, and arm reaches.

- Focus on keeping your core engaged and your body centered over the pad.

- Start with simple movements and gradually increase the difficulty by adding dynamic or asymmetrical movements.

3. **Stability Ball Exercises**:

- Sit on a stability ball with your feet flat on the ground and your knees bent at a 90-degree angle.

- Engage your core and lift one foot off the ground, balancing on the stability ball.

- Hold the position for 10-30 seconds, then switch feet.

- To progress, try lifting both feet off the ground or incorporating upper body movements such as arm circles or overhead reaches.

4. **Agility Ladder Drills**:

- Set up an agility ladder on the ground.

- Perform a variety of agility drills, such as high knees, lateral shuffles, and crossover steps, by stepping in and out of the ladder rungs with speed and precision.

- Focus on quick footwork, coordination, and maintaining balance as you move through the drills.

- Start with simple patterns and progress to more complex combinations as your skills improve.

5. **Tai Chi or Qigong**:

- Practice Tai Chi or Qigong, ancient Chinese martial arts that emphasize slow, flowing movements, mindfulness, and breath control.

- Perform gentle, choreographed sequences of movements that incorporate balance, coordination, and relaxation techniques.

- Focus on maintaining smooth, continuous movements and connecting your breath with each movement.

- Tai Chi and Qigong are suitable for all ages and fitness levels and can be practiced indoors or outdoors.

6. **Yoga Balancing Poses**:

- Incorporate balancing yoga poses into your practice, such as Tree Pose, Warrior III, and Half Moon Pose.

- Stand tall with your feet hip-width apart and shift your weight onto one leg.

- Slowly lift the opposite foot off the ground and place the sole of your foot against your inner thigh, calf, or ankle, avoiding the knee joint.

- Find a focal point to gaze at and engage your core to maintain balance.

- Hold the pose for 30-60 seconds, then switch sides.

Integrating Balance and Coordination into Daily Life

In addition to specific exercises, here are some practical tips for integrating balance and coordination into your daily routine:

1. Mindful Movement: Practice mindful movement throughout the day by paying attention to your posture, alignment, and movement patterns. Focus on moving with intention,

awareness, and precision in everything you do, from walking and standing to reaching and bending.

2. **Multisensory Training**: Challenge your balance and coordination by exposing yourself to different sensory stimuli and environmental conditions. Practice balance exercises with your eyes closed, on unstable surfaces, or while performing dual tasks to enhance proprioception and neuromuscular control.

3. **Functional Training**: Emphasize functional training exercises that mimic real-life movement patterns and

activities. Choose exercises that require a combination of balance, coordination, strength, and flexibility to support everyday activities and sports performance.

4. **Progressive Overload**: Gradually increase the difficulty and complexity of your balance and coordination exercises as your skills improve. Start with simple movements and progress to more challenging variations, such as adding dynamic or asymmetrical movements, increasing the speed or duration of the exercises, or performing them on unstable surfaces.

5. **Consistency and Patience**: Be consistent in your practice of balance and coordination exercises, but also be patient and realistic in your expectations. Improving balance and coordination takes time, dedication, and consistent effort, so stay committed to your practice and trust in the process.

Unveiling the Essence of Balance

Before delving into the strategies, it's essential to uncover the essence of balance and why it's vital for overall well-being:

1. Foundation of Movement: Balance forms the foundation upon which all movement is built. It allows us to stand tall,

walk with confidence, and navigate our surroundings with ease.

2. **Core Stability**: Balance training strengthens the core muscles, including the abdominals, obliques, and lower back, which play a pivotal role in stabilizing the body and maintaining proper posture.

3. **Injury Prevention:** Improving balance reduces the risk of falls and injuries by enhancing proprioception, coordination, and neuromuscular control. By training the body to adapt to changes in position and terrain, we can move with greater confidence and resilience.

Strategies for Integrating Balance Training into your Routine

Now, let's explore practical strategies for incorporating balance training into your routine:

1. Start Small and Progress Gradually:

Begin with simple balance exercises that challenge your stability without overwhelming your body. Start by standing on one leg for a few seconds at a time, then gradually increase the duration as your balance improves. As you gain confidence, progress to more challenging exercises, such as standing on unstable surfaces or performing dynamic movements.

2. Incorporate Balance into Everyday Activities:

Look for opportunities to integrate balance training into your daily routine. Practice standing on one leg while brushing your teeth, waiting in line, or cooking dinner. Incorporate balance challenges into household chores by standing on a balance board while folding laundry or washing dishes. By incorporating balance into everyday activities, you can improve stability and coordination without setting aside dedicated workout time.

3. Utilize Balance Equipment

Invest in balance equipment such as stability balls, balance boards, wobble cushions, and foam pads to add variety to your workouts and challenge your balance in different ways. Experiment with different surfaces and textures to target different muscle groups and enhance proprioception. Incorporate balance equipment into your strength training, yoga, or Pilates routine to improve stability and coordination while building strength and flexibility.

4. Practice Mindful Movement

Approach balance training with mindfulness and intention, focusing on the sensations in your body and the quality of your movement. Pay attention to your breath, posture, and alignment as you perform balance exercises, and cultivate a sense of presence and awareness in each moment. Mindful movement not only enhances the effectiveness of your training but also promotes relaxation, stress relief, and overall well-being.

5. Challenge Yourself

Don't be afraid to step outside your comfort zone and challenge yourself with new and unfamiliar balance exercises. Try balancing on one leg with your eyes closed, performing dynamic movements on an unstable surface, or incorporating balance challenges into your strength training routine. By pushing your limits and exploring new movement patterns, you can improve proprioception, coordination, and neuromuscular control while building confidence and resilience.

6. Be Consistent

Consistency is key when it comes to balance training. Aim to incorporate balance exercises into your routine at least 2-3 times per week to see results. Set aside dedicated time for balance training, whether it's during your workout sessions, before or after your regular exercise routine, or as part of your warm-up or cool-down. By making balance training a regular part of your routine, you can improve stability, coordination, and overall movement quality over time.

Practical Balance Training Exercises

Now, let's explore some practical balance training exercises that you can incorporate into your routine:

1. Single-Leg Stance

Stand tall with your feet hip-width apart.

Shift your weight onto one leg and lift the opposite foot off the ground, balancing on the standing leg.

Engage your core and maintain a tall posture as you hold the position for 30-60 seconds.

Switch legs and repeat on the opposite side.

To progress, try closing your eyes or performing arm movements while balancing.

2. Stability Ball Knee Tucks

Start in a plank position with your hands on the ground and your shins resting on a stability ball.

Engage your core and lift your hips to form a straight line from your head to your heels.

Maintaining balance, bend your knees and pull the stability ball towards your chest, then extend your legs to return to the starting position.

Repeat for 10-15 repetitions, focusing on maintaining stability and control throughout the movement.

3. Bosu Ball Squats

Stand on a Bosu ball with your feet hip-width apart and your core engaged.

Lower into a squat position, keeping your weight

in your heels and your knees tracking over your toes.

Maintain your balance as you lower down and press back up to the starting position.

Repeat for 10-15 repetitions, focusing on maintaining stability and control throughout the movement.

4. Single-Leg Deadlifts

Stand tall with your feet hip-width apart and your arms at your sides.

Shift your weight onto one leg and hinge forward at the hips, extending your opposite leg behind you for balance.

Keep your back flat and your core engaged as you lower your torso towards the ground, reaching your hands towards your standing foot.

Pause briefly at the bottom, then return to the starting position by squeezing your glutes and driving through your standing heel.

Repeat for 10-15 repetitions on each leg, focusing on maintaining stability and control throughout the movement.

5. **Yoga Tree Pose**

Stand tall with your feet hip-width apart and your arms at your sides.

Shift your weight onto one foot and lift the opposite foot off the ground, placing the sole of your foot against your inner thigh, calf, or ankle.

Press your foot into your leg and your leg into your foot to create stability, then bring your hands together at your heart center.

Find a focal point to gaze at to help maintain balance, then hold the pose for 30-60 seconds.

Switch sides and repeat on the opposite leg, focusing on maintaining stability and control throughout the pose.

Chapter 7

Habit 6 - Posture Alignment Practices Understanding the Importance of Proper Posture

In the symphony of movement, proper posture serves as the conductor, orchestrating harmony, balance, and alignment throughout the body. Chapter 7 delves into the realm of posture alignment practices, shedding light on the significance of maintaining proper posture for overall health and well-being. From understanding the impact of posture on physical and mental health to practical strategies for improving alignment, we explore the keys to unlocking greater vitality, confidence, and resilience through posture awareness.

The Foundations of Posture

Before delving into the importance of proper posture, let's establish a foundational understanding of what posture is and why it matters:

1. **Definition:** Posture refers to the alignment and positioning of the body's joints, muscles, and bones in

relation to one another. It encompasses the way we stand, sit, walk, and move throughout the day.

2. **Alignment:** Proper posture involves maintaining a neutral alignment of the spine, pelvis, shoulders, and hips, with minimal strain or tension on the muscles and joints. It allows for optimal distribution of weight and support of the body's structures.

3. **Function**: Good posture supports efficient movement patterns, optimal organ function, and overall well-being. It helps to prevent muscle imbalances, joint dysfunction, and pain, while promoting stability, balance, and energy efficiency.

The Importance of Proper Posture

Now, let's explore why proper posture is crucial for overall health and well-being:

1. **Spinal Health**: Proper posture helps to maintain the natural curves of the spine, including the cervical (neck), thoracic (mid-back), and lumbar (lower back) regions. It reduces the risk of spinal misalignment, disc compression, and nerve impingement, which can lead to back pain, stiffness, and dysfunction.

2. **Musculoskeletal Health**: Good posture promotes balanced muscle development and optimal joint alignment, reducing the risk of muscle imbalances, joint strain, and overuse injuries. It supports efficient movement patterns and prevents excessive wear and tear on the muscles, ligaments, and tendons.

3. **Breathing and Digestion:** Proper posture allows for optimal lung expansion and diaphragmatic breathing, enhancing respiratory function and oxygen delivery to the body's tissues. It also supports proper alignment of the digestive organs, promoting efficient digestion and nutrient absorption.

4. **Balance and Stability**: Maintaining proper posture improves balance, stability, and proprioception, reducing the risk of falls and injuries, especially as we age. It enhances coordination, spatial awareness, and neuromuscular control, supporting safe and efficient movement in various activities of daily living.

5. **Mental Health**: Good posture has been linked to improved mood, confidence, and self-esteem. It promotes a sense of openness, presence, and assertiveness, while reducing feelings of stress, tension, and fatigue. By standing

tall and confident, we project an image of strength and vitality to the world around us.

Practical Strategies for Improving Posture

Now that we understand the importance of proper posture, let's explore practical strategies for improving alignment and posture awareness:

1. **Posture Awareness**:

- Start by developing awareness of your posture throughout the day. Notice how you stand, sit, walk, and move, and observe any habits or tendencies that may contribute to poor posture.

- Pay attention to the alignment of your spine, pelvis, shoulders, and hips, and make adjustments as needed to maintain proper posture.

- Use mirrors, video recordings, or posture apps to monitor your posture and track your progress over time.

2. **Ergonomic Environment**:

- Create an ergonomic environment at home and work to support good posture. Choose supportive furniture, such as ergonomic chairs and desks, that promote neutral spine alignment and proper body positioning.

- Adjust your workstation to optimize ergonomics, including the height of your chair, the position of your computer monitor, and the placement of your keyboard and mouse.

- Take regular breaks to stretch, move, and reset your posture throughout the day, especially if you spend long periods sitting or standing.

3. Core Strengthening:

- Strengthen the core muscles, including the abdominals, obliques, and lower back, to support proper posture and spinal alignment.

- Incorporate core-strengthening exercises into your routine, such as planks, bridges, bird dogs, and Russian twists, to build stability and strength in the torso.

- Focus on engaging the core muscles during daily activities to maintain stability and support proper posture.

4. Stretching and Mobility:

- Incorporate stretching and mobility exercises into your routine to release tension, improve flexibility, and enhance posture.

- Focus on areas of tightness or restriction, such as the chest, shoulders, hips, and hamstrings, and perform dynamic and static stretches to increase range of motion and relieve muscular tension.

- Practice yoga, Pilates, or mobility drills to improve joint mobility, spinal flexibility, and overall posture alignment.

5. Mindful Movement:

- Practice mindful movement throughout the day by paying attention to your posture, alignment, and movement patterns.

- Focus on standing tall with your shoulders back and down, your chin tucked, and your core engaged. Imagine a string pulling you upward from the top of your head, lengthening your spine and creating space between each vertebra.

- Cultivate a sense of presence and awareness in each moment, and notice how your posture affects your mood, energy levels, and overall well-being.

Embracing the Journey of Posture Alignment

In conclusion, proper posture is essential for supporting optimal health, well-being, and vitality. By understanding the importance of posture and implementing practical strategies for improving alignment and posture awareness, we can enhance spinal health, musculoskeletal function, and overall quality of life. So let us embrace the journey of posture alignment with curiosity, dedication, and a commitment to nurturing our body's innate wisdom and vitality.

Correcting Common Postural Imbalances

In the intricate dance of movement, posture serves as the silent conductor, orchestrating harmony, balance, and alignment throughout the body. Chapter 7 delves into the realm of posture alignment practices, focusing on correcting common postural imbalances. From understanding the root causes of postural deviations to practical strategies for restoring balance and alignment, we explore the keys to unlocking greater vitality, confidence, and resilience through posture awareness and corrective exercises.

Unraveling the Web of Postural Imbalances

Before delving into corrective strategies, it's crucial to understand the common postural imbalances that can occur:

1. Forward Head Posture: This occurs when the head juts forward from its neutral position, often due to prolonged sitting, poor posture habits, or excessive screen time. Forward head posture can lead to neck pain, headaches, and cervical spine dysfunction.

2. **Rounded Shoulders**: Rounded shoulders result from tightness in the chest muscles and weakness in the upper back muscles, causing the shoulders to slump forward. This can be exacerbated by poor posture, hunching over electronic devices, or improper lifting techniques.

3. **Anterior Pelvic Tilt:** Anterior pelvic tilt occurs when the pelvis tilts forward, causing the lower back to arch excessively and the abdomen to protrude. This imbalance is often associated with tight hip flexors, weak glutes, and prolonged sitting, leading to lower back pain and hip dysfunction.

4. **Swayback Posture**: Swayback posture is characterized by an exaggerated curvature of the spine, with the pelvis tilted forward and the upper back rounded. It can result from a combination of factors, including weak core muscles, tight hip flexors, and poor postural habits, leading to back pain and spinal misalignment.

The Importance of Correcting Postural Imbalances

Now, let's explore why it's essential to correct postural imbalances:

1. Pain Relief: Correcting postural imbalances can alleviate chronic pain and discomfort, particularly in the neck,

shoulders, back, and hips. By restoring proper alignment and balance, we can reduce the strain on muscles and joints, leading to improved comfort and mobility.

2. Injury Prevention: Addressing postural imbalances can help prevent injuries by reducing the risk of overuse, strain, and repetitive stress. By improving alignment and movement patterns, we can enhance the body's ability to withstand physical stressors and maintain optimal function.

3. **Improved Function**: Correcting postural imbalances enhances functional movement patterns, allowing us to move with greater efficiency, stability, and range of motion. By restoring balance and alignment, we can perform everyday activities with ease and confidence, from walking and standing to lifting and reaching.

4. Enhanced Performance: Proper posture is essential for optimal athletic performance, as it allows for efficient movement mechanics, power generation, and coordination. By addressing postural imbalances, athletes can improve their strength, speed, and agility, leading to better sports performance and reduced risk of injury.

Practical Strategies for Correcting Postural Imbalances

Now that we understand the importance of correcting postural imbalances, let's explore practical strategies for restoring balance and alignment:

1. Stretching Tight Muscles:

- Focus on stretching tight muscles that contribute to postural imbalances, such as the chest, shoulders, hip flexors, and hamstrings.

- Incorporate dynamic and static stretches into your routine to improve flexibility and release tension in these areas.

- Hold each stretch for 20-30 seconds and repeat several times on each side, focusing on slow, controlled movements and deep breathing.

2. Strengthening Weak Muscles:

- Target weak muscles that contribute to postural imbalances, such as the upper back, core, glutes, and deep abdominal muscles.

- Perform strengthening exercises that target these areas, such as rows, reverse flyes, planks, bridges, squats, and lunges.

- Gradually increase the intensity and difficulty of these exercises as your strength improves, focusing on proper form and alignment.

3. **Postural Awareness and Correction**:

- Develop awareness of your posture throughout the day and make conscious efforts to correct any imbalances.

- Practice standing tall with your shoulders back and down, your chin tucked, and your core engaged. Imagine a string pulling you upward from the top of your head, lengthening your spine and creating space between each vertebra.

- Use mirrors, video recordings, or posture apps to monitor your posture and track your progress over time. Make adjustments as needed to maintain proper alignment and balance.

4. **Ergonomic Environment**:

- Create an ergonomic environment at home and work to support good posture. Choose supportive furniture, such as ergonomic chairs and desks, that promote neutral spine alignment and proper body positioning.

- Adjust your workstation to optimize ergonomics, including the height of your chair, the position of your computer monitor, and the placement of your keyboard and mouse.

- Take regular breaks to stretch, move, and reset your posture throughout the day, especially if you spend long periods sitting or standing.

5. Functional Movement Training:

- Incorporate functional movement training into your routine to improve mobility, stability, and coordination.

- Perform exercises that mimic real-life movement patterns, such as squats, lunges, hinges, and rotations, to reinforce balanced movement patterns and support functional performance.

- Focus on maintaining proper alignment and control throughout each movement, and progress gradually as you build strength and confidence.

Embracing the Journey of Postural Alignment and resilience.

Implementing Posture Alignment Techniques into Your Daily Life

In the rhythm of our everyday lives, the significance of posture often remains unnoticed, relegated to a mere afterthought amidst the hustle and bustle. Yet, within the intricate tapestry of our bodies, posture serves as the silent conductor, orchestrating balance, harmony, and alignment. It's the foundation upon which we build our physical and emotional well-being, influencing everything from our confidence and presence to our overall health and vitality.

The Foundations of Posture Alignment

Before we dive into the nitty-gritty of posture alignment techniques, let's first understand the fundamentals of good posture. Posture alignment refers to the optimal positioning of the body's joints, muscles, and bones in relation to one another, allowing for efficient movement and balanced distribution of weight. When our posture is aligned, we experience less strain on our muscles and joints, reducing the risk of pain, injury, and fatigue.

Good posture encompasses several key elements:

1. **Alignment**: The spine should maintain its natural curves, with the head aligned over the shoulders and the pelvis in a

neutral position. The shoulders should be relaxed and level, not rounded or hunched forward.

2. **Balance**: The body should be evenly balanced over its base of support, with weight distributed evenly between the feet. This promotes stability and reduces the risk of falls or injury.

3. **Engagement**: Core muscles, including the abdominals and lower back muscles, should be engaged to support the spine and pelvis and maintain proper alignment.

4.**Awareness**: Developing awareness of your posture throughout the day allows you to make conscious adjustments and prevent slouching or poor alignment habits.

The Benefits of Good Posture

The benefits of good posture extend far beyond mere aesthetics. Maintaining proper alignment has numerous physical, mental, and emotional benefits, including:

- **Reduced Pain and Discomfort**: Good posture helps alleviate strain on muscles and joints, reducing the risk of chronic pain, tension headaches, and musculoskeletal disorders.

- **Improved Breathing and Circulation**: Proper alignment allows for optimal lung expansion and blood flow, enhancing oxygen delivery to the brain and muscles and promoting overall vitality.

- **Enhanced Confidence and Presence**: Standing tall with good posture conveys confidence, poise, and authority, making a positive impression on others and boosting self-esteem.

- **Better Digestion and Digestive Health**: Good posture supports proper alignment of the digestive organs, facilitating digestion and reducing the risk of gastrointestinal issues such as acid reflux or constipation.

- **Increased Energy and Productivity:** Maintaining good posture reduces fatigue and improves energy levels, allowing you to stay focused, alert, and productive throughout the day.

Integrating Posture Alignment Techniques into Your Daily Routine

Now that we understand the importance of good posture, let's explore practical strategies for integrating posture alignment techniques into your daily life:

1. **Mindful Awareness**:

- Start by developing mindfulness of your body's alignment throughout the day. Notice how you sit, stand, and move, and make conscious adjustments to improve your posture.

- Set reminders on your phone or computer to check in with your posture regularly, especially during prolonged periods of sitting or standing.

2. **Ergonomic Environment**:

- Create an ergonomic workstation that supports good posture. Ensure that your chair provides adequate lumbar support and that your desk is at the correct height to promote neutral wrist and elbow alignment.

- Adjust your computer monitor so that it is at eye level, reducing strain on your neck and shoulders.

3. **Core Strengthening**:

- Incorporate core-strengthening exercises into your fitness routine to support good posture. Exercises such as planks, bridges, and bird-dogs target the muscles that help stabilize the spine and pelvis.

- Practice engaging your core muscles throughout the day, especially during activities that require lifting or bending.

4. **Stretching and Mobility**:

- Perform regular stretching exercises to improve flexibility and release tension in tight muscles that can contribute to poor posture. Focus on stretching the chest, shoulders, hip flexors, and hamstrings.

- Incorporate mobility exercises into your routine to improve joint range of motion and reduce stiffness. Gentle movements such as shoulder circles, hip circles, and spinal twists can help maintain healthy joint function.

5. **Posture Alignment Exercises:**

- Practice specific posture alignment exercises to reinforce proper alignment and address common postural imbalances.

Exercises such as chin tucks, shoulder retractions, and pelvic tilts can help realign the spine and improve posture.

- Consider incorporating mind-body practices such as yoga or Pilates into your routine, as these disciplines emphasize body awareness, alignment, and breath control.

6. Mindful Movement:

- Pay attention to how you move throughout the day, focusing on maintaining proper alignment and avoiding slouching or awkward positions. Practice walking with purpose, standing tall, and moving with grace and intention.

- Experiment with mindful movement practices such as tai chi or qigong, which promote fluidity, balance, and alignment through slow, deliberate movements.

Chapter 8

Habit 7 - Mobility Nutrition Nourishing Your Body for Optimal Mobility

In the pursuit of optimal mobility, we often focus on physical activity, stretching, and strengthening exercises. However, one crucial aspect of mobility that is sometimes overlooked is nutrition. Just as fuel is essential for a car to run smoothly, the food we consume plays a fundamental role in supporting our body's mobility and overall health. In this chapter, we will explore the importance of mobility nutrition and discover how nourishing your body with the right foods can enhance your flexibility, strength, and resilience.

Understanding Mobility Nutrition:

1. **Fueling Your Body**: Think of your body as a finely-tuned machine, requiring the right balance of nutrients to function optimally. Just as a car needs fuel to operate, your body needs a combination of carbohydrates, proteins, fats, vitamins, and minerals to support mobility and physical performance.

2. **Nutrient-Rich Foods**: Focus on consuming nutrient-dense foods that provide essential vitamins, minerals, and antioxidants to support joint health, muscle function, and tissue repair. Include a variety of fruits, vegetables, whole grains, lean proteins, and healthy fats in your diet to ensure you're getting a broad spectrum of nutrients.

3. **Hydration**: Proper hydration is essential for maintaining joint lubrication, regulating body temperature, and supporting cellular function. Drink plenty of water throughout the day, and consider adding electrolyte-rich beverages such as coconut water or sports drinks during intense physical activity to replenish lost fluids and minerals.

4. **Anti-Inflammatory Foods**: Chronic inflammation can contribute to joint stiffness, pain, and reduced mobility. Incorporate anti-inflammatory foods such as fatty fish (e.g., salmon, mackerel), nuts, seeds, olive oil, turmeric, ginger, and leafy greens into your diet to help reduce inflammation and support joint health.

5. **Protein for Muscle Repair**: Protein is essential for muscle repair and recovery, especially after exercise. Include lean sources of protein such as chicken, turkey, fish, tofu,

beans, and lentils in your meals to support muscle growth and repair.

6. **Healthy Fats:** Omega-3 fatty acids found in fatty fish, flaxseeds, chia seeds, and walnuts have anti-inflammatory properties and support joint health. Incorporate these healthy fats into your diet to help reduce inflammation and promote mobility.

7. **Bone Health**: Calcium, vitamin D, and magnesium are essential nutrients for maintaining strong and healthy bones. Include calcium-rich foods such as dairy products, leafy greens, and fortified foods, as well as vitamin D-rich foods such as fatty fish, eggs, and fortified dairy alternatives to support bone health and prevent fractures.

8. **Flexibility and Mobility**: Certain nutrients, such as vitamin C and collagen, play a role in supporting connective tissue health and flexibility. Include vitamin C-rich foods such as citrus fruits, bell peppers, and strawberries, as well as collagen-rich foods such as bone broth, chicken skin, and fish skin in your diet to support joint flexibility and mobility.

Practical Strategies for Mobility Nutrition:

1. **Meal Planning**: Plan and prepare meals in advance to ensure you have healthy, nutritious options readily available.

Focus on incorporating a variety of nutrient-rich foods into your meals, including fruits, vegetables, whole grains, lean proteins, and healthy fats.

2. **Balanced Meals**: Aim to create balanced meals that include a combination of carbohydrates, proteins, and fats to provide sustained energy and support muscle repair and recovery. Include colorful fruits and vegetables, lean proteins, whole grains, and healthy fats in each meal to ensure you're getting a broad spectrum of nutrients.

3. **Snack Smart:** Choose nutrient-dense snacks such as fresh fruit, vegetables with hummus or nut butter, Greek yogurt, or nuts and seeds to keep your energy levels stable and support muscle recovery between meals.

4. **Hydration**: Drink water throughout the day to stay hydrated and support joint lubrication and cellular function. Aim to drink at least 8-10 cups of water per day, and adjust your fluid intake based on your activity level and environmental conditions.

5. **Pre- and Post-Workout Nutrition**: Fuel your body with a combination of carbohydrates and protein before and after exercise to support energy levels, muscle repair, and recovery. Choose easily digestible snacks such as a banana with nut butter or Greek yogurt with berries before exercise,

and a protein-rich snack such as a protein shake or chocolate milk after exercise to refuel and repair muscles.

6. **Supplementation**: Consider supplementing your diet with vitamins and minerals that support joint health and mobility, such as glucosamine, chondroitin, omega-3 fatty acids, and vitamin D. Consult with a healthcare professional or registered dietitian to determine if supplementation is right for you and to ensure you're taking appropriate doses.

7. **Mindful Eating**: Practice mindful eating by paying attention to hunger and fullness cues, eating slowly, and savoring the flavors and textures of your food. Avoid distractions such as TV or screens while eating, and listen to your body's signals to determine when you're hungry and when you're satisfied.

8. **Consistency**: Consistency is key when it comes to mobility nutrition. Make healthy eating a habit by incorporating nutritious foods into your daily routine and making mindful choices that support your overall health and well-being.

Incorporating Mobility Nutrition into Your Lifestyle

1. **Start Small**: Begin by making small changes to your diet, such as adding an extra serving of vegetables to your meals

or swapping out sugary snacks for healthier alternatives. Gradually build on these changes over time to create a sustainable, nutrient-rich eating pattern.

2. **Set Goals**: Set specific, measurable goals for improving your nutrition and mobility, such as increasing your daily intake of fruits and vegetables, drinking more water, or reducing your consumption of processed foods. Track your progress and celebrate your achievements along the way to stay motivated and focused on your goals.

3. **Seek Support**: Surround yourself with a supportive network of friends, family, or health professionals who can provide encouragement, accountability, and guidance as you work towards improving your nutrition and mobility. Share your goals with others and enlist their support in helping you stay on track.

4. **Stay Flexible**: Remember that nutrition is not one-size-fits-all, and what works for one person may not work for another. Stay flexible and open-minded as you explore different dietary approaches and find what works best for your body and lifestyle.

5. **Listen to Your Body**: Pay attention to how different foods make you feel and adjust your diet accordingly. Experiment

with different foods and eating patterns to find what makes you feel energized, satisfied, and nourished.

Foods That Promote Joint Health and Flexibility

In the quest for optimal mobility and flexibility, the role of nutrition cannot be overstated. While exercise and stretching are essential components of a healthy lifestyle, the foods we consume play a crucial role in supporting joint health, reducing inflammation, and enhancing flexibility. In this chapter, we explore the power of nutrition in promoting joint health and flexibility, and identify key foods that can help you move with greater ease and comfort.

Understanding Joint Health and Flexibility:

Before delving into the specific foods that promote joint health and flexibility, let's first understand the importance of these two aspects of mobility.

1. **Joint Health**: Joints are the points where two or more bones meet, allowing for movement and flexibility. Maintaining healthy joints is crucial for overall mobility and functionality, as well as for preventing conditions such as arthritis, stiffness, and pain.

2. **Flexibility**: Flexibility refers to the range of motion of a joint or group of joints. Good flexibility allows for smooth and unrestricted movement, reducing the risk of injury and improving performance in physical activities.

Nutrients That Support Joint Health and Flexibility:

Several nutrients play a key role in supporting joint health and flexibility. Incorporating these nutrients into your diet can help promote mobility, reduce inflammation, and support overall joint function. Some of the most important nutrients include:

1. **Omega-3 Fatty Acids**: Omega-3 fatty acids are essential fats that have anti-inflammatory properties and are critical for maintaining joint health. Fatty fish such as salmon, mackerel, and sardines are rich sources of omega-3s, as are flaxseeds, chia seeds, and walnuts.

2. **Vitamin D**: Vitamin D is essential for calcium absorption and bone health, both of which are crucial for maintaining strong and healthy joints. Sunlight is the primary source of vitamin D, but it can also be found in foods such as fatty fish, egg yolks, and fortified dairy products.

3. **Vitamin C**: Vitamin C is an antioxidant that plays a role in collagen synthesis, which is essential for maintaining the

structure and function of joints and connective tissues. Citrus fruits, strawberries, bell peppers, and kiwi are excellent sources of vitamin C.

4. **Collagen:** Collagen is the most abundant protein in the body and is a key component of cartilage, tendons, and ligaments. Consuming collagen-rich foods such as bone broth, chicken skin, and fish skin can help support joint health and flexibility.

5. **Antioxidants:** Antioxidants help protect the body from oxidative stress and inflammation, both of which can contribute to joint pain and stiffness. Colorful fruits and vegetables such as berries, cherries, spinach, and kale are rich sources of antioxidants.

6. **Calcium and Magnesium**: Calcium and magnesium are essential minerals for bone health and muscle function, both of which are important for maintaining joint health and flexibility. Dairy products, leafy greens, nuts, seeds, and whole grains are good sources of calcium and magnesium.

Foods That Promote Joint Health and Flexibility

Now that we understand the importance of these nutrients, let's explore some specific foods that can help promote joint health and flexibility:

1. **Fatty Fish**: Fatty fish such as salmon, mackerel, and sardines are rich sources of omega-3 fatty acids, which have anti-inflammatory properties and are essential for joint health. Aim to include fatty fish in your diet at least two to three times per week.

2. **Leafy Greens**: Leafy greens such as spinach, kale, and collard greens are packed with vitamins, minerals, and antioxidants that support joint health and flexibility. Add leafy greens to salads, smoothies, soups, and stir-fries for an extra boost of nutrition.

3. **Berries**: Berries such as blueberries, strawberries, and raspberries are rich in antioxidants, particularly vitamin C, which plays a role in collagen synthesis and joint health. Enjoy berries as a snack, add them to yogurt or oatmeal, or blend them into smoothies for a delicious and nutritious treat.

4. **Nuts and Seeds**: Nuts and seeds are excellent sources of omega-3 fatty acids, as well as calcium, magnesium, and antioxidants. Include nuts and seeds such as walnuts, almonds, flaxseeds, and chia seeds in your diet as a healthy snack or as toppings for salads, yogurt, or oatmeal.

5. **Bone Broth**: Bone broth is rich in collagen, gelatin, and amino acids that support joint health and flexibility. Enjoy bone broth as a warm and comforting beverage, or use it as a base for soups, stews, and sauces.

6. **Turmeric:** Turmeric is a spice that contains curcumin, a compound with powerful anti-inflammatory and antioxidant properties. Add turmeric to soups, curries, stir-fries, and smoothies to reap its joint-protective benefits.

7. **Yogurt**: Yogurt is a rich source of calcium and vitamin D, both of which are important for bone health and joint function. Choose plain, unsweetened yogurt and add your own toppings such as fresh fruit, nuts, and seeds for a nutritious and satisfying snack.

8. **Avocado**: Avocado is a nutrient-dense fruit that is rich in healthy fats, vitamins, minerals, and antioxidants. Enjoy avocado sliced on toast, added to salads, or blended into smoothies for a creamy and nutritious boost.

Incorporating These Foods into Your Diet

Now that we've identified some key foods that promote joint health and flexibility, let's explore practical strategies for incorporating these foods into your diet:

1. **Meal Planning**: Plan your meals and snacks in advance to ensure you're getting a variety of nutrient-rich foods throughout the day. Include a mix of fatty fish, leafy greens, berries, nuts, seeds, and other joint-friendly foods in your meal plan.

2. **Recipe Ideas**: Explore new recipes that incorporate these joint-friendly foods in creative and delicious ways. Look for recipes for salmon salads, kale smoothies, chia seed puddings, and turmeric-spiced dishes to add variety to your diet.

3. **Healthy Swaps**: Make healthy swaps in your favorite recipes to include more joint-friendly foods. For example, swap out regular pasta for spiralized zucchini noodles, or use Greek yogurt instead of sour cream in dips and dressings.

4 **snack Smart**: Keep a selection of healthy snacks on hand that include joint-friendly foods such as nuts, seeds, yogurt, and fresh fruit. Choose nutrient-dense snacks that provide sustained energy and support joint health throughout the day.

5. **Hydration**: Remember to stay hydrated by drinking plenty of water throughout the day. Hydration is important

for joint lubrication, muscle function, and overall health, so aim to drink at least 8-10 cups of water per day.

Nutrition Strategies for Supporting Overall Mobility

In our pursuit of optimal mobility, we often focus on physical activity, stretching, and strengthening exercises. However, nutrition plays a critical role in supporting overall mobility and flexibility. The foods we consume provide the building blocks for healthy joints, muscles, and connective tissues, while also supplying the energy needed for movement and physical activity. In this chapter, we will explore nutrition strategies specifically tailored to support overall mobility, enhancing our ability to move freely and comfortably through life.

Understanding Mobility Nutrition:

Before diving into specific nutrition strategies, it's essential to understand the key nutrients that support overall mobility and flexibility:

1. **Protein**: Protein is essential for muscle repair and growth, which is crucial for maintaining strength and flexibility. Including adequate protein in your diet ensures that your muscles have the necessary building blocks to recover from exercise and daily activities.

2. **Omega-3 Fatty Acids**: Omega-3 fatty acids have anti-inflammatory properties and play a role in reducing joint pain and stiffness. Consuming foods rich in omega-3s can help support joint health and mobility, reducing the risk of inflammation-related mobility issues.

3. **Antioxidants**: Antioxidants help protect cells from damage caused by free radicals, which can contribute to inflammation and joint degeneration. Eating a diet rich in antioxidants from fruits, vegetables, and other plant-based foods can help support overall joint health and mobility.

4. **Hydration**: Proper hydration is essential for maintaining joint lubrication and flexibility. Drinking an adequate amount of water throughout the day ensures that your joints stay well-hydrated and can move smoothly without discomfort.

5. **Vitamins and Minerals**: Certain vitamins and minerals, such as vitamin D, calcium, and magnesium, play a role in bone health and muscle function, both of which are important for overall mobility. Including a variety of nutrient-rich foods in your diet ensures that you get the vitamins and minerals needed to support mobility.

Now that we understand the key nutrients that support overall mobility, let's explore some nutrition strategies for incorporating these nutrients into our diet:

1. **Focus on Whole Foods**: Fill your plate with whole, nutrient-dense foods such as fruits, vegetables, lean proteins, whole grains, and healthy fats. These foods provide essential vitamins, minerals, and antioxidants that support overall mobility and health.

2. **Include Protein with Every Meal**: Aim to include a source of protein with every meal and snack to support muscle repair and growth. Good sources of protein include lean meats, poultry, fish, eggs, dairy products, legumes, nuts, and seeds.

3. **Incorporate Omega-3-Rich Foods:** Include omega-3-rich foods such as fatty fish (salmon, mackerel, sardines), flaxseeds, chia seeds, walnuts, and hemp seeds in your diet regularly to support joint health and reduce inflammation.

4. **Eat Plenty of Fruits and Vegetables**: Fruits and vegetables are rich in antioxidants, vitamins, and minerals that support overall health and mobility. Aim to fill half your plate with colorful fruits and vegetables at each meal to ensure you get a variety of nutrients.

5. **Stay Hydrated**: Drink plenty of water throughout the day to stay hydrated and support joint lubrication. Aim to drink at least 8-10 cups of water per day, or more if you are active or live in a hot climate.

6. **Limit Processed Foods and Added Sugars**: Processed foods and added sugars can contribute to inflammation and joint pain. Limit your intake of processed foods, sugary beverages, and snacks high in added sugars, and focus on whole, minimally processed foods instead.

7. **Include Calcium-Rich Foods**: Calcium is essential for bone health and muscle function, both of which are important for overall mobility. Include calcium-rich foods such as dairy products, leafy greens, tofu, and fortified plant-based milk alternatives in your diet regularly.

8. **Get Plenty of Vitamin D**: Vitamin D plays a role in calcium absorption and bone health, both of which are important for overall mobility. Get vitamin D from sunlight exposure and include vitamin D-rich foods such as fatty fish, egg yolks, and fortified dairy products in your diet.

Practical Nutrition Tips for Supporting Overall Mobility

Now that we've covered some general nutrition strategies for supporting overall mobility, let's explore some practical tips for incorporating these strategies into your daily routine:

1. **Plan Balanced Meals**: Plan your meals ahead of time to ensure they include a balance of protein, carbohydrates, and healthy fats, along with plenty of fruits and vegetables. Batch cooking and meal prepping can help save time and ensure you have healthy meals ready to go throughout the week.

2. **Keep Healthy Snacks on Hand**: Stock your pantry and fridge with healthy snacks such as fresh fruit, vegetables with hummus, Greek yogurt, nuts, and seeds. Having healthy snacks on hand makes it easier to make nutritious choices when hunger strikes between meals.

3. **Experiment with New Recipes**: Explore new recipes and cooking techniques to keep meals interesting and enjoyable. Look for recipes that incorporate a variety of nutrient-rich foods and flavors to keep your taste buds satisfied.

4. **Stay Mindful of Portions**: Pay attention to portion sizes to avoid overeating and support a healthy weight. Use measuring cups, spoons, and food scales to measure portions, especially when trying new foods or recipes.

5. **Listen to Your Body**: Pay attention to how different foods make you feel and adjust your diet accordingly. Notice how your energy levels, mood, and overall well-being are affected by the foods you eat, and make changes as needed to support optimal mobility and health.

6. **Stay Consistent**: Consistency is key when it comes to nutrition and overall mobility. Make healthy eating a habit by incorporating nutritious foods into your daily routine and making mindful choices that support your goals.

7. **Seek Support**: Don't be afraid to seek support from a registered dietitian or nutritionist if you need help navigating nutrition and overall mobility. A qualified professional can provide personalized guidance and support to help you reach your health and fitness goals.

Chapter 9

Recovery and Regeneration
The Role of Recovery in Enhancing Mobility

In our fast-paced modern world, we often push ourselves to the limit, constantly striving for improvement and achievement. However, in our pursuit of progress, we often overlook the importance of rest, recovery, and regeneration. In this chapter, we explore the critical role of recovery in enhancing mobility, optimizing performance, and preventing injury. We delve into the science of recovery, uncovering the physiological processes that occur during rest, and explore practical strategies for incorporating recovery techniques into our daily lives.

Understanding Recovery and Regeneration

Before diving into specific recovery techniques, it's essential to understand the concept of recovery and its significance in the context of mobility and performance.

1. Definition of Recovery: Recovery refers to the process of restoring the body to a state of balance and homeostasis after exercise or physical activity. It encompasses various physiological and psychological processes that occur during

rest, including muscle repair, glycogen replenishment, hormone regulation, and central nervous system recovery.

2. **Importance of Recovery**: Recovery is essential for optimizing performance, preventing injury, and supporting overall health and well-being. Adequate recovery allows the body to repair damaged tissues, replenish energy stores, and adapt to the stress of exercise, leading to improvements in strength, endurance, and mobility.

3. **Types of Recovery**: There are several types of recovery, including passive recovery (resting without engaging in physical activity), active recovery (engaging in low-intensity exercise or movement), and specific recovery modalities such as stretching, foam rolling, massage, compression therapy, and cold therapy.

Now that we understand the importance of recovery let's explore the specific ways in which recovery techniques can enhance mobility:

1. **Muscle Repair and Regeneration**: Intense physical activity, such as strength training or high-intensity interval training, can cause microscopic damage to muscle fibers. During recovery, the body repairs and rebuilds these damaged muscle fibers, leading to increases in muscle strength, size, and flexibility.

2. **Glycogen Replenishment**: Glycogen is the primary fuel source for muscles during exercise, and depletion of glycogen stores can lead to fatigue and decreased performance. During recovery, the body replenishes glycogen stores in the muscles and liver, ensuring that energy reserves are fully restored for future physical activity.

3. **Hormone Regulation**: Exercise can alter hormone levels in the body, including cortisol, testosterone, and growth hormone. Adequate recovery helps regulate these hormone levels, promoting muscle growth, fat loss, and overall metabolic health.

4. **Central Nervous System Recovery:** Intense exercise can stress the central nervous system, leading to fatigue and reduced coordination. Recovery allows the central nervous system to recover, improving neuromuscular function, coordination, and mobility.

5. **Injury Prevention**: Recovery techniques such as stretching, foam rolling, and massage can help prevent injuries by improving flexibility, reducing muscle tension, and enhancing joint mobility. Incorporating these techniques into your routine can help maintain optimal mobility and reduce the risk of overuse injuries.

Practical Strategies for Recovery and Regeneration

Now that we understand the importance of recovery let's explore some practical strategies for incorporating recovery techniques into our daily lives:

1. **Rest and Sleep**: Adequate rest and sleep are essential for recovery and regeneration. Aim for 7-9 hours of quality sleep per night, and prioritize rest days in your training schedule to allow your body to recover from intense physical activity.

2. **Hydration:** Proper hydration is crucial for recovery, as it helps transport nutrients to the muscles and remove metabolic waste products. Drink plenty of water throughout the day, and consider consuming electrolyte-rich beverages such as coconut water or sports drinks during and after exercise to replenish lost fluids and minerals.

3. **Nutrition:** Nutrition plays a critical role in recovery, providing the building blocks for muscle repair and glycogen replenishment. Consume a balanced diet that includes a mix of carbohydrates, proteins, and healthy fats, and prioritize nutrient-dense foods such as fruits, vegetables, lean proteins, whole grains, and healthy fats.

4. **Active Recovery**: Incorporate active recovery activities such as walking, cycling, swimming, or yoga into your routine on rest days or after intense workouts. Low-intensity exercise helps improve blood flow, reduce muscle soreness,

and promote recovery without causing additional stress on the body.

5. **Stretching and Mobility Work**: Include stretching, mobility exercises, and foam rolling in your recovery routine to improve flexibility, reduce muscle tension, and enhance joint mobility. Focus on targeting tight or sore muscles, and hold stretches for 30-60 seconds to allow for maximum muscle relaxation and lengthening.

6. **Massage and Bodywork**: Treat yourself to regular massages or bodywork sessions to help release muscle tension, improve circulation, and promote relaxation. Alternatively, invest in a foam roller, massage ball, or massage gun for self-myofascial release at home.

7. **Compression Therapy**: Consider using compression garments or compression therapy devices to enhance recovery by improving circulation, reducing inflammation, and speeding up the removal of metabolic waste products from the muscles.

8. **Cold Therapy:** Take advantage of cold therapy techniques such as ice baths, cold showers, or cryotherapy to reduce inflammation, numb sore muscles, and accelerate recovery. Apply cold packs or ice packs to sore or injured

areas for 10-20 minutes at a time to help reduce pain and swelling.

Incorporating Recovery Techniques into Your Routine:

Now that we've explored some practical strategies for recovery and regeneration let's explore how to incorporate these techniques into your routine:

1. **Schedule Recovery Days**: Plan rest days into your training schedule to allow your body to recover from intense workouts. Use these days to focus on passive recovery activities such as rest, relaxation, and gentle movement.

2. **Prioritize Sleep**: Make sleep a priority by establishing a consistent sleep schedule, creating a relaxing bedtime routine, and optimizing your sleep environment for restful sleep. Aim for 7-9 hours of quality sleep per night to support recovery and regeneration.

3. **Listen to Your Body**: Pay attention to how your body feels and adjust your training intensity, volume, and

frequency accordingly. If you're feeling fatigued or sore, consider taking a rest day or engaging in low-intensity activities to promote recovery.

4. **Plan Active Recovery Sessions**: Incorporate active recovery activities such as walking, cycling, swimming, or yoga into your routine on rest days or after intense workouts. These activities help improve blood flow, reduce muscle soreness, and promote relaxation without causing additional stress on the body.

5. **Make Time for Stretching and Mobility Work**: Set aside time each day to perform stretching, mobility exercises, and foam rolling to improve flexibility, reduce muscle tension, and enhance joint mobility. Focus on targeting tight or sore muscles, and hold stretches for 30-60 seconds to allow for maximum muscle relaxation and lengthening.

6. **Schedule Massage or Bodywork Sessions**: Treat yourself to regular massages or bodywork sessions to help release muscle tension, improve circulation, and promote relaxation. Alternatively, invest in a foam roller, massage ball, or massage gun for self-myofascial release at home.

7. **Use Compression Therapy**: Incorporate compression garments or compression therapy devices into your recovery routine to enhance circulation, reduce inflammation, and speed up recovery. Wear compression garments during or

after workouts, or use compression therapy devices for targeted compression and recovery.

8. **Try Cold Therapy**: Experiment with cold therapy techniques such as ice baths, cold showers, or cryotherapy to reduce inflammation, numb sore muscles, and accelerate recovery. Apply cold packs or ice packs to sore or injured areas for 10-20 minutes at a time to help reduce pain and swelling.

Techniques for Effective Muscle Recovery

Recovery is an essential component of any fitness regimen, yet it's often overlooked or undervalued in favor of intense workouts and pushing physical limits. However, without adequate recovery, the body can't adapt, grow stronger, or perform at its best. In this chapter, we delve into the art of muscle recovery, exploring various techniques and strategies to help you recover effectively and optimize your performance.

Understanding Muscle Recovery

Before diving into specific techniques, let's understand what muscle recovery entails and why it's crucial for overall fitness and well-being.

1. **Definition of Muscle Recovery**: Muscle recovery refers to the process by which the body repairs and rebuilds muscle fibers that have been damaged during exercise. This process involves various physiological mechanisms, including protein synthesis, glycogen replenishment, and tissue repair.

2. **Importance of Muscle Recovery**: Muscle recovery is essential for several reasons:

- It allows muscles to repair and rebuild, leading to muscle growth and strength gains.

- It replenishes energy stores, such as glycogen, which are depleted during exercise.

- It reduces the risk of injury by giving the body time to repair damaged tissues and recover from fatigue.

- It allows the central nervous system to recover, improving coordination and motor skills.

Now that we understand the importance of muscle recovery, let's explore some techniques to help you recover effectively:

1. **Rest and Sleep**

- Adequate rest and sleep are fundamental for muscle recovery. During sleep, the body releases growth hormone, which promotes muscle repair and growth.

- Aim for 7-9 hours of quality sleep per night, and prioritize rest days in your training schedule to allow your muscles time to recover.

2. **Nutrition**

- Nutrition plays a critical role in muscle recovery, providing the necessary nutrients for tissue repair and growth.

- Consume a balanced diet rich in lean proteins, complex carbohydrates, healthy fats, vitamins, and minerals.

- Aim to consume a post-workout meal or snack containing protein and carbohydrates to replenish energy stores and support muscle repair.

3. **Hydration**

- Proper hydration is essential for muscle recovery, as dehydration can impair performance and delay recovery.

- Drink plenty of water throughout the day, and consider consuming electrolyte-rich beverages during and after exercise to replace lost fluids and minerals.

4. **Active Recovery** - Engaging in light physical activity on rest days can help promote blood flow, reduce muscle soreness, and enhance recovery.

- Activities such as walking, cycling, swimming, or yoga can serve as effective forms of active recovery.

5. Stretching and Foam Rolling:

- Stretching and foam rolling can help alleviate muscle tension, improve flexibility, and promote recovery.

- Incorporate dynamic stretches before exercise to warm up the muscles and static stretches after exercise to cool down and prevent stiffness.

- Use a foam roller or massage ball to target tight or sore muscles and release trigger points.

6. Massage Therapy

- Massage therapy can help relieve muscle tension, reduce soreness, and improve circulation, promoting faster recovery.

- Consider scheduling regular massage sessions with a licensed massage therapist or using self-massage techniques such as self-myofascial release with a foam roller or massage ball.

7. Compression Garments

- Compression garments, such as compression socks or sleeves, can help improve circulation, reduce muscle vibration, and enhance recovery.

- Wear compression garments during or after exercise to support muscle recovery and reduce post-exercise soreness.

8. Cold Therapy

- Cold therapy, such as ice baths or cold showers, can help reduce inflammation, numb sore muscles, and speed up recovery.

- Apply ice packs or cold packs to sore or inflamed areas for 10-20 minutes at a time to help alleviate pain and swelling.

9. Heat Therapy:

- Heat therapy, such as warm baths or heating pads, can help relax muscles, increase blood flow, and promote recovery.

- Apply heat to tight or sore muscles for 15-20 minutes at a time to help reduce muscle tension and improve mobility.

Incorporating Muscle Recovery Techniques into Your Routine:

Now that we've explored various muscle recovery techniques, let's discuss how to incorporate them into your routine:

1. Create a Recovery Plan:

- Develop a structured recovery plan that includes rest days, active recovery activities, and recovery techniques such as stretching, foam rolling, and massage therapy.

- Schedule recovery sessions into your weekly training schedule and prioritize them as you would any other workout.

2. Listen to Your Body:

- Pay attention to how your body feels and adjust your training intensity, volume, and frequency accordingly.

- If you're feeling fatigued or sore, consider taking a rest day or engaging in light physical activity to promote recovery.

3. Experiment with Different Techniques: - Try different muscle recovery techniques to see which ones work best for you.

- Experiment with stretching, foam rolling, massage therapy, compression garments, and cold therapy to find the combination that helps you recover most effectively.

4. **Be Consistent**:

- Consistency is key when it comes to muscle recovery. Make recovery a regular part of your routine, rather than an afterthought.

- Incorporate recovery techniques into your daily or weekly routine and stick with them to maximize their benefits.

5. **Prioritize Sleep and Nutrition**:

- Prioritize sleep and nutrition as integral components of muscle recovery.

- Aim for 7-9 hours of quality sleep per night, and consume a balanced diet rich in lean proteins, complex carbohydrates, healthy fats, vitamins, and minerals to support muscle repair and growth.

Prioritizing Rest and Regeneration for Long-Term Mobility

In our fast-paced world filled with demanding schedules and endless distractions, the value of rest and recovery often gets overshadowed. However, if we truly want to achieve long-term mobility and overall well-being, we must recognize the critical role that rest and regeneration play in our fitness journey. In this chapter, we delve into the importance of prioritizing rest and regeneration for long-term mobility, exploring why it matters and how we can integrate it into our lives.

Understanding Rest and Regeneration

Before delving into the specifics, let's first understand what rest and regeneration entail and why they are crucial for long-term mobility.

1. **Rest:** Rest refers to the act of abstaining from physical exertion or mental stress. It's a period of relaxation and recovery during which the body and mind have the opportunity to recharge and repair.

2. **Regeneration**: Regeneration encompasses the processes by which the body restores and rejuvenates itself. This includes muscle repair, tissue rebuilding, hormone regulation, and mental recovery.

Now that we've defined rest and regeneration, let's explore why they are essential for long-term mobility:

1. **Muscle Repair and Growth**: During rest, the body repairs and rebuilds muscle fibers that have been damaged

during exercise. This process is essential for muscle recovery, growth, and adaptation to training stimuli.

2. **Energy Replenishment**: Rest allows the body to replenish energy stores such as glycogen, which are depleted during physical activity. Adequate energy reserves are necessary for sustained performance and optimal mobility.

3. **Hormone Regulation**: Rest plays a crucial role in hormone regulation, including the release of growth hormone, testosterone, and cortisol. These hormones influence muscle repair, recovery, and overall metabolic function.

4. **Mental Recovery**: Rest is not only essential for physical recovery but also for mental recovery. It provides an opportunity to relax, unwind, and recharge mentally, reducing stress and enhancing overall well-being.

Now that we understand the importance of rest and regeneration let's explore some strategies for prioritizing them in our lives:

1. **Schedule Regular Rest Days**

   - Incorporate rest days into your weekly training schedule to allow your body time to recover from intense workouts.

Aim for at least one or two rest days per week, depending on your fitness level and training intensity.

2. Listen to Your Body:

- Pay attention to how your body feels and adjust your training intensity, volume, and frequency accordingly. If you're feeling fatigued or sore, it may be a sign that you need more rest.

3. Prioritize Sleep:

- Sleep is essential for rest and regeneration, as it allows the body to repair and rejuvenate itself. Aim for 7-9 hours of quality sleep per night, and prioritize sleep hygiene practices such as maintaining a consistent sleep schedule, creating a relaxing bedtime routine, and optimizing your sleep environment.

4. Practice Mindfulness and Relaxation Techniques:

- Incorporate mindfulness and relaxation techniques into your daily routine to reduce stress and promote mental recovery. Techniques such as deep breathing, meditation, yoga, and progressive muscle relaxation can help calm the mind and promote restful sleep.

5. Nourish Your Body

- Proper nutrition is essential for rest and regeneration, as it provides the necessary nutrients for muscle repair and energy replenishment. Consume a balanced diet rich in whole foods such as fruits, vegetables, lean proteins, whole grains, and healthy fats.

6. **Hydrate Adequately**:

- Hydration is crucial for rest and regeneration, as dehydration can impair recovery and performance. Drink plenty of water throughout the day, and consider consuming electrolyte-rich beverages during and after exercise to replace lost fluids and minerals.

7. **Incorporate Active Recovery**:

- Engage in light physical activity on rest days to promote blood flow, reduce muscle soreness, and enhance recovery. Activities such as walking, cycling, swimming, or gentle yoga can serve as effective forms of active recovery.

8. **Prioritize Mental Health**:

- Mental health is an integral component of rest and regeneration. Make time for activities that bring you joy, relaxation, and fulfillment, whether it's spending time with loved ones, pursuing hobbies, or practicing self-care.

Incorporating Rest and Regeneration into Your Routine:

Now that we've explored some strategies for prioritizing rest and regeneration let's discuss how to incorporate them into your daily life:

1. **Plan Your Rest Days**

   - Schedule rest days into your weekly calendar and treat them as non-negotiable appointments. Use this time to relax, recharge, and engage in activities that promote rest and recovery.

2. **Establish a Bedtime Routine**:

   - Create a relaxing bedtime routine to signal to your body that it's time to wind down and prepare for sleep. This may include activities such as reading, taking a warm bath, or practicing relaxation techniques.

3. **Set Boundaries**:

   - Learn to set boundaries and prioritize your own needs when it comes to rest and regeneration. Don't be afraid to say no to activities or commitments that interfere with your rest and recovery time.

4. **Practice Self-Compassion**   - Be kind to yourself and recognize that rest is a vital part of the fitness journey. Avoid

guilt or self-criticism for taking rest days and prioritize your long-term health and well-being.

5. Monitor Your Progress

- Keep track of your rest and recovery practices and monitor how they impact your mobility, performance, and overall well-being. Adjust your approach as needed based on your observations and feedback from your body.

Chapter 10

Habit 9 - Mind-Body Connection
Harnessing the Power of Mindfulness for Mobility

In the pursuit of mobility and physical fitness, we often focus solely on the body—training muscles, stretching ligaments, and strengthening joints. However, we tend to overlook the crucial role that the mind plays in our physical capabilities. The mind-body connection is a powerful force that can greatly influence our mobility, flexibility, and overall well-being. In this chapter, we delve into the concept of mindfulness and explore how harnessing the power of mindfulness can enhance our mobility and enrich our lives.

Understanding the Mind-Body Connection:

Before diving into mindfulness, let's first understand the concept of the mind-body connection and why it's essential for mobility:

1. Definition of Mind-Body Connection: The mind-body connection refers to the intricate relationship between the mind and the body, wherein mental processes and emotions

influence physical health and vice versa. This connection emphasizes the holistic nature of human beings, recognizing that mental and emotional states can impact physical well-being.

2. **Importance of the Mind-Body Connection**: The mind-body connection is essential for overall health and well-being, including mobility, flexibility, and physical performance. By cultivating awareness of our thoughts, emotions, and sensations, we can better understand and respond to the needs of our bodies, leading to improved movement patterns, reduced risk of injury, and enhanced overall mobility.

Now that we understand the importance of the mind-body connection let's explore how mindfulness can help harness this power for mobility:

1. **Definition of Mindfulness**:

- Mindfulness is the practice of paying attention to the present moment with openness, curiosity, and acceptance. It involves bringing awareness to our thoughts, emotions, sensations, and surroundings without judgment or attachment.

2. **Benefits of Mindfulness for Mobility** - Mindfulness can have profound effects on mobility and physical performance:

- Increased Body Awareness: Mindfulness helps cultivate a greater sense of body awareness, allowing us to tune into subtle sensations, movement patterns, and areas of tension or imbalance.

- Enhanced Movement Quality: By bringing mindful awareness to our movements, we can improve movement quality, efficiency, and coordination, leading to smoother, more fluid motion.

- Reduced Stress and Tension: Mindfulness practices such as deep breathing, meditation, and body scanning can help reduce stress, tension, and muscular tightness, promoting relaxation and ease of movement.

- Improved Mental Focus: Mindfulness enhances mental focus and concentration, allowing us to stay present and engaged during physical activities, leading to better performance and reduced risk of injury.

- Enhanced Mind-Body Integration: By cultivating mindfulness, we can strengthen the connection between the mind and body, enabling us to move with greater intention, control, and precision.

- Faster Recovery: Mindfulness practices such as meditation and visualization can help promote faster recovery by reducing inflammation, improving sleep quality, and enhancing overall well-being.

Practical Strategies for Cultivating Mindfulness for Mobility:

Now that we understand the benefits of mindfulness for mobility, let's explore some practical strategies for incorporating mindfulness into our daily lives:

1. **Mindful Movement Practices**:

- Engage in mindful movement practices such as yoga, tai chi, qigong, or Pilates, which emphasize awareness of breath, movement, and body sensations. These practices can help improve flexibility, balance, and mobility while promoting relaxation and stress reduction.

2. **Body Scan Meditation**:

- Practice body scan meditation to cultivate awareness of bodily sensations and promote relaxation. Start by focusing your attention on different parts of your body, scanning from head to toe, and noticing any sensations, tension, or areas of discomfort. Allow yourself to breathe into these sensations and let go of any tension or tightness.

3. **Breath Awareness**:

- Develop a regular breath awareness practice to anchor your attention in the present moment and calm the mind. Practice mindful breathing exercises such as deep belly breathing, diaphragmatic breathing, or square breathing to promote relaxation, reduce stress, and enhance focus.

4. **Mindful Walking**:

- Practice mindful walking by bringing awareness to each step, sensation, and movement of your body as you walk. Notice the sensation of your feet touching the ground, the rhythm of your breath, and the sights and sounds around you. Walking mindfully can help ground you in the present moment and promote a sense of calm and presence.

5. **Visualization Techniques**:

- Use visualization techniques to enhance mobility and performance by mentally rehearsing movements, sequences, or activities. Visualize yourself moving with ease, fluidity, and precision, imagining each movement in vivid detail.

Visualization can help improve motor skills, confidence, and mind-body coordination.

6. Mindful Eating:

- Practice mindful eating by bringing awareness to the sensory experience of eating, including the taste, texture, and aroma of food. Slow down and savor each bite, chewing mindfully and paying attention to hunger and satiety cues. Mindful eating can help promote healthier eating habits, digestion, and overall well-being.

Incorporating Mindfulness into Your Daily Routine:

Now that we've explored practical strategies for cultivating mindfulness for mobility let's discuss how to incorporate these practices into your daily routine:

1. Create a Daily Mindfulness Practice

- Set aside dedicated time each day for mindfulness practice, whether it's in the morning, during lunch breaks, or before bedtime. Start with just a few minutes and gradually increase the duration as you build your practice.

2. Integrate Mindfulness into Daily Activities:

- Look for opportunities to incorporate mindfulness into your daily activities, such as brushing your teeth, washing dishes, or walking to work. Use these moments as opportunities to bring awareness to your breath, body sensations, and surroundings.

3. **Use Reminders and Cues**:

- Use reminders and cues to help you remember to practice mindfulness throughout the day. Set alarms on your phone, place sticky notes in visible locations, or link mindfulness practices to existing habits or routines.

4. **Practice Gratitude and Mindful Reflection**:

- Take time each day to reflect on what you're grateful for and cultivate a sense of appreciation for the present moment. Notice the beauty and wonder in everyday experiences, and express gratitude for the blessings in your life.

5. **Find Support and Accountability**:

- Seek out support and accountability from friends, family members, or mindfulness communities. Share your experiences, challenges, and insights with others who share your interest in mindfulness and mobility.

Mental Techniques for Enhancing Physical Mobility

In the realm of physical mobility, the mind often takes a backseat to the body. However, the mind-body connection is a powerful force that can greatly influence our physical capabilities. Our thoughts, beliefs, and mental processes can profoundly impact our movement patterns, flexibility, and overall mobility. In this chapter, we explore the importance of the mind-body connection and delve into mental techniques that can enhance physical mobility.

Understanding the Mind-Body Connection

The mind-body connection refers to the intricate relationship between our thoughts, emotions, and physical sensations. This connection highlights the interplay between mental and physical states, emphasizing the holistic nature of human beings. Here are some key aspects of the mind-body connection:

1. **Awareness**: Developing awareness of our thoughts, emotions, and physical sensations is essential for understanding the mind-body connection. By tuning into our internal experiences, we can recognize patterns, triggers, and areas of tension or discomfort.

2. **Intention:** Our intentions and motivations shape our actions and behaviors. By setting clear intentions and aligning them with our physical goals, we can harness the power of the mind to enhance our mobility and performance.

3. **Beliefs**: Our beliefs and attitudes about ourselves and our bodies influence our perception of our physical abilities. Positive beliefs can boost confidence, motivation, and resilience, while negative beliefs can hinder performance and limit potential.

4. **Visualization**: Visualization is a powerful mental technique that involves imagining ourselves performing movements or activities with precision and skill. By mentally rehearsing movements, we can enhance motor learning, coordination, and confidence.

5. **Mindfulness:** Mindfulness is the practice of being present and attentive to our thoughts, emotions, and sensations without judgment. By cultivating mindfulness, we can deepen our awareness of the mind-body connection and enhance our ability to regulate our physical responses.

Now that we understand the mind-body connection let's explore some mental techniques for enhancing physical mobility:

1. **Setting Clear Intentions**:

Setting clear intentions is the first step toward enhancing physical mobility. Whether it's improving flexibility, mastering a new movement, or recovering from an injury, clarity of intention provides direction and focus. Take some time to reflect on your goals and aspirations for your mobility journey, and set specific, achievable intentions that align with your values and priorities.

2. **Practicing Positive Self-Talk**

Our internal dialogue has a profound impact on our self-perception and physical capabilities. Positive self-talk involves replacing negative or self-limiting thoughts with affirming, empowering statements. Instead of saying, "I can't do this," try saying, "I am capable and resilient." Cultivate a mindset of self-compassion, resilience, and confidence, and watch how it transforms your approach to mobility and movement.

3. **Visualizing Success**

Visualization is a powerful tool for enhancing physical performance. Take time each day to visualize yourself performing movements with ease, grace, and precision. Imagine yourself moving fluidly, confidently, and effortlessly, achieving your mobility goals with ease. Visualization primes the mind and body for success, enhancing motor learning, coordination, and confidence.

4. Practicing Mindful Movement

Mindful movement involves bringing awareness to our movements, sensations, and breath as we engage in physical activities. Whether it's yoga, tai chi, or simply walking, practice moving with intention, presence, and curiosity. Notice the sensations in your body, the rhythm of your breath, and the subtle shifts in your posture and alignment. Mindful movement enhances proprioception, body awareness, and coordination, leading to improved mobility and performance.

5. Using Breathwork for Relaxation and Focus

Breathwork is a powerful tool for calming the mind, reducing stress, and enhancing focus. Practice deep breathing exercises such as diaphragmatic breathing, square breathing, or alternate nostril breathing to promote relaxation and concentration. Use breathwork techniques to center yourself before engaging in physical activities, and notice how it enhances your mobility, flexibility, and overall well-being.

6. **Cultivating Resilience and Adaptability**:

The journey toward enhanced physical mobility is not always smooth sailing. It's important to cultivate resilience and adaptability in the face of challenges and setbacks. Instead of viewing obstacles as roadblocks, see them as opportunities for growth and learning. Approach your mobility journey with a mindset of curiosity, experimentation, and perseverance, knowing that every setback is a stepping stone toward greater resilience and mastery.

7.**Practicing Gratitude and Mindfulness:**

Gratitude and mindfulness are powerful practices for enhancing the mind-body connection and promoting overall well-being. Take time each day to cultivate gratitude for your body and its incredible capacity for movement and expression. Practice mindfulness by bringing awareness to the present moment, savoring the sensations of movement, and appreciating the gift of mobility.

Incorporating Mental Techniques into Your Mobility Routine Now that we've explored some mental techniques for enhancing physical mobility let's discuss how to incorporate them into your daily routine:

1. Set aside dedicated time for mental training:

Schedule regular time each day for mental training and practice. Whether it's a few minutes of visualization before bed or a mindful movement practice in the morning, prioritize your mental well-being as you would your physical training.

2. Integrate mental techniques into your workouts

Incorporate mental techniques such as visualization, positive self-talk, and breathwork into your workouts and training sessions. Use them to enhance focus, motivation, and performance, and notice how they impact your physical capabilities.

3. Stay consistent and patient:

Like any skill, mental techniques require practice and patience to master. Stay consistent with your practice, even when progress feels slow or elusive. Trust in the process and remain open to the possibilities that arise from cultivating a strong mind-body connection.

4. Seek support and guidance

Don't hesitate to seek support and guidance from mentors, coaches, or mental health professionals who can help you develop and refine your mental techniques. Share your experiences, challenges, and insights with others who share your interest in enhancing physical mobility through mental training.

Cultivating a Strong Mind-Body Connection

In the pursuit of physical fitness and mobility, we often focus solely on the body, neglecting the profound influence of the mind on our movement and overall well-being. However, the mind-body connection is a powerful force that can significantly impact our physical capabilities, performance, and quality of life. Cultivating a strong mind-body connection involves developing awareness, intention, and alignment between our mental and physical states. In this chapter, we delve into the importance of the mind-body connection and explore practical strategies for nurturing and strengthening this vital relationship.

Understanding the Mind-Body Connection

The mind-body connection refers to the intricate interplay between our thoughts, emotions, and physical sensations. It recognizes the inseparable link between mental processes and bodily functions, highlighting the holistic nature of human beings. Here are some key aspects of the mind-body connection:

1. **Awareness**: Developing awareness of our thoughts, emotions, and physical sensations is the foundation of the mind-body connection. By tuning into our internal experiences, we can gain insight into the relationship between our mental and physical states.

2. **Intention**: Intention refers to the conscious direction of our thoughts and actions toward a specific goal or outcome. Setting clear intentions aligns our mental and physical efforts, guiding us toward greater coherence and integration.

3. **Beliefs:** Our beliefs and attitudes about ourselves and our bodies shape our perception of reality and influence our behavior. Positive beliefs can enhance confidence, motivation, and resilience, while negative beliefs can limit potential and hinder performance.

4. **Breath**: Breath is a powerful bridge between the mind and body, serving as a conduit for energy, awareness, and presence. Cultivating conscious breathing practices can help

regulate the nervous system, reduce stress, and enhance mind-body integration.

5. Movement: Movement is an expression of our inner state, reflecting our thoughts, emotions, and intentions. Mindful movement practices such as yoga, tai chi, and qigong emphasize the connection between breath, body, and mind, fostering greater awareness and embodiment.

Now that we understand the components of the mind-body connection, let's explore practical strategies for cultivating a strong and resilient connection:

1. Developing Awareness:

The first step in cultivating a strong mind-body connection is developing awareness of our internal experiences. This involves paying attention to our thoughts, emotions, and physical sensations without judgment or attachment. Mindfulness practices such as meditation, body scanning, and breath awareness can help sharpen our awareness and deepen our understanding of the mind-body connection.

2. Setting Clear Intentions:

Setting clear intentions aligns our mental and physical efforts toward a specific goal or outcome. Whether it's improving mobility, enhancing performance, or promoting relaxation, clarity of intention provides direction and focus. Take time to reflect on your values and priorities, and set intentions that resonate with your deepest aspirations.

3. Practicing Positive Affirmations:

Positive affirmations are empowering statements that reinforce positive beliefs and self-perceptions. By repeating affirmations such as "I am strong," "I am resilient," or "I am capable," we can rewire our subconscious mind and cultivate a more positive and supportive internal dialogue. Incorporate affirmations into your daily routine to boost confidence, motivation, and self-esteem.

4. Engaging in Mindful Movement:

Mindful movement practices such as yoga, tai chi, and qigong emphasize the integration of breath, body, and mind. These practices promote greater awareness, presence, and embodiment, fostering a deep sense of connection between our internal and external worlds. Explore different forms of mindful movement and find practices that resonate with your body and spirit.

5. Practicing Breathwork

Breathwork is a powerful tool for regulating the nervous system, reducing stress, and enhancing mind-body coherence. Explore different breathing techniques such as diaphragmatic breathing, box breathing, or alternate nostril breathing to cultivate a deeper connection with your breath. Incorporate breathwork into your daily routine to promote relaxation, focus, and vitality.

6. Cultivating Gratitude

Cultivating gratitude is a potent practice for shifting our perspective and fostering a deeper appreciation for life. Take time each day to reflect on the blessings in your life and express gratitude for your body and its incredible capacity for movement and expression. Cultivating an attitude of gratitude can enhance resilience, optimism, and overall well-being.

7. Nurturing Self-Compassion

Self-compassion is the practice of extending kindness, understanding, and acceptance to ourselves, especially in times of difficulty or challenge. Treat yourself with the same kindness and compassion you would offer to a dear friend, and recognize that you are worthy of love and care. Nurturing self-compassion fosters a deeper sense of connection and acceptance, strengthening the mind-body connection.

Incorporating Mind-Body Practices into Your Daily Life

Now that we've explored practical strategies for cultivating a strong mind-body connection, let's discuss how to incorporate these practices into your daily life:

1. Create Daily Rituals

Establish daily rituals that support your mind-body connection, such as morning meditation, mindful movement sessions, or evening reflection practices. Set aside dedicated time each day for self-care and introspection, and prioritize your well-being as a non-negotiable aspect of your routine.

2. Integrate Mindfulness into Daily Activities

Infuse mindfulness into your daily activities by bringing awareness to the present moment. Whether you're eating, walking, or engaging in household chores, practice being fully present and attentive to your experience. Notice the sensations in your body, the rhythm of your breath, and the beauty of the world around you.

Cultivate Supportive Environments:

Surround yourself with people and environments that support your mind-body connection and well-being. Seek out communities, classes, or groups that share your values and interests, and cultivate meaningful connections with like-minded individuals. Create a supportive environment at home and work that nurtures your growth and development.

4. Embrace Challenges as Opportunities for Growth

View challenges and setbacks as opportunities for growth and learning. Instead of resisting or avoiding difficult experiences, approach them with curiosity and openness, knowing that they offer valuable lessons and insights. Cultivate resilience and adaptability in the face of adversity, and trust in your ability to navigate life's ups and downs with grace and wisdom.

5. Practice Patience and Persistence:

Cultivating a strong mind-body connection is a journey that requires patience, persistence, and self-compassion. Be gentle with yourself as you explore new practices and navigate the complexities of your inner landscape. Trust in the process of growth and transformation, and know that every step you take brings you closer to greater harmony and integration.

Chapter 11

Habit 10 - Lifelong Learning and Adaptability

Embracing a Growth Mindset for Lifelong Mobility

In the journey towards lifelong mobility and vitality, one of the most critical habits we can cultivate is a growth mindset. This mindset involves embracing challenges, persisting in the face of setbacks, and continuously seeking opportunities for learning and growth. By adopting a growth mindset, we open ourselves up to new possibilities, expand our capabilities, and navigate life's ups and downs with resilience and optimism. In this chapter, we explore the importance of lifelong learning and adaptability for mobility and vitality and provide practical strategies for embracing a growth mindset.

Understanding the Growth Mindset

A growth mindset is a belief system that focuses on the potential for growth and development throughout life. Individuals with a growth mindset view challenges as opportunities for learning, setbacks as temporary obstacles, and failure as a natural part of the learning process. They believe that with effort, perseverance, and the right strategies, they can improve their skills, abilities, and overall quality of life.

1. Embracing Challenges

People with a growth mindset embrace challenges as opportunities to stretch their abilities and expand their horizons. Instead of shying away from difficulty, they welcome it as a chance to learn, grow, and improve.

2. Persisting in the Face of Adversity:

A growth mindset enables individuals to persevere in the face of adversity. Rather than giving up when faced with obstacles, they view setbacks as temporary setbacks and remain resilient in their pursuit of their goals.

3. Seeking Opportunities for Learning and Growth:

Individuals with a growth mindset are always on the lookout for opportunities to learn and grow. They seek out new experiences, challenges, and feedback, knowing that each presents an opportunity for personal and professional development.

4. **Learning from Failure**: Failure is seen as a natural part of the learning process for those with a growth mindset. Instead of letting failure discourage them, they use it as a learning opportunity, extracting valuable lessons and insights that they can apply to future endeavors.

5. **Cultivating Curiosity**: A growth mindset is characterized by a sense of curiosity and wonder about the world. People with this mindset are eager to explore new ideas, try new things, and push the boundaries of what they thought possible.

Now that we understand the components of a growth mindset let's explore practical strategies for embracing lifelong learning and adaptability for mobility and vitality:

1. **Set Learning Goals**: Set specific, achievable goals for your learning and personal development. Whether it's mastering a new skill, exploring a new hobby, or pursuing further education, having clear goals gives you direction and motivation to keep moving forward.

2. **Develop a Growth-Oriented Mindset**:

Cultivate a mindset that embraces growth and development. Instead of viewing your abilities as fixed, believe that with effort and perseverance, you can improve and grow over time. Focus on progress rather than perfection, and celebrate your achievements along the way.

3. **Challenge Yourself Regularly**:

Step out of your comfort zone and challenge yourself to try new things. Whether it's taking on a new project at work, learning a new language, or trying a new form of exercise, pushing yourself beyond your limits helps you grow and develop new skills and abilities.

4. **Seek Feedback and Learn from Mistakes:**

Actively seek out feedback from others and be open to constructive criticism. Use feedback as an opportunity to learn and improve, and don't be afraid to make mistakes along the way. Remember that failure is not a reflection of your abilities but a stepping stone on the path to success.

5. **Cultivate Resilience and Persistence:** Cultivate resilience and persistence in the face of challenges and setbacks. When things don't go as planned, don't give up. Instead, learn from the experience, adjust your approach, and keep moving forward with determination and optimism.

6. **Stay Curious and Open-Minded**:

Cultivate a sense of curiosity and open-mindedness about the world around you. Stay curious about new ideas, perspectives, and experiences, and be open to learning from others. Approach life with a sense of wonder and excitement, and never stop asking questions.

Incorporating Lifelong Learning and Adaptability into Your Life

Now that we've explored practical strategies for embracing a growth mindset let's discuss how to incorporate these habits into your daily life:

1. **Make Learning a Priority:**

Make learning a priority in your life by setting aside dedicated time for personal and professional development. Whether it's reading books, taking online courses, or attending workshops and seminars, invest in yourself and your growth on a regular basis.

2. **Surround Yourself with Lifelong Learners**

Surround yourself with people who share your commitment to lifelong learning and personal growth. Seek out mentors, coaches, and peers who inspire and challenge you to be your best self, and learn from their wisdom and experience.

3. Stay Flexible and Adapt to Change

Embrace change as a natural part of life and stay flexible and adaptable in the face of uncertainty. Instead of resisting change, see it as an opportunity for growth and transformation, and approach new challenges with curiosity and optimism.

4. Reflect on Your Learning Journey

Take time to reflect on your learning journey and celebrate your progress and achievements. Keep a journal or reflective log where you can document your experiences, insights, and lessons learned along the way.

5. Share Your Knowledge and Experience

Share your knowledge and experience with others and contribute to the collective growth and development of your community. Whether it's mentoring a colleague, teaching a class, or volunteering your time and expertise, find ways to give back and pay it forward.

Continual Learning and Adaptation for Mobility

In the pursuit of lifelong mobility and vitality, there exists a fundamental truth: the journey never truly ends. Our bodies, minds, and circumstances are in a perpetual state of change, requiring us to continually learn, adapt, and evolve in order to maintain our mobility and well-being. This chapter explores the importance of continual learning and adaptation for mobility and vitality, providing insights and strategies for embracing a mindset of growth and resilience throughout life's journey.

Understanding the Need for Continual Learning and Adaptation

Life is dynamic and ever-changing, presenting us with new challenges, opportunities, and experiences at every turn. In order to thrive in this constantly evolving landscape, we must cultivate a mindset of continual learning and adaptation. Here are some key reasons why continual learning and adaptation are essential for mobility:

1. Changing Needs and Abilities:

As we age, our bodies undergo various changes that can affect our mobility and physical capabilities. From changes in muscle mass and bone density to shifts in joint mobility and flexibility, our bodies require ongoing attention and adaptation to maintain optimal function.

2. Advancements in Knowledge and Technology

The fields of health, fitness, and mobility are constantly evolving, with new research, techniques, and technologies emerging on a regular basis. In order to stay abreast of the latest developments and innovations, we must commit to lifelong learning and professional development.

3. Environmental and Lifestyle Factors

Our mobility and vitality are also influenced by environmental factors such as our living and working environments, as well as our lifestyle choices and habits. By continually learning and adapting to our surroundings, we can optimize our mobility and well-being in the face of changing circumstances.

4. Personal Growth and Fulfillment

Finally, continual learning and adaptation are essential for personal growth and fulfillment. By challenging ourselves to learn new skills, explore new interests, and overcome new challenges, we can expand our horizons, build resilience, and experience greater fulfillment in our lives.

Now that we understand the importance of continual learning and adaptation let's explore practical strategies for embracing this mindset for mobility and vitality:

1. Stay Curious and Open-Minded

Cultivate a sense of curiosity and open-mindedness about the world around you. Approach life with a sense of wonder and excitement, and never stop asking questions or seeking out new experiences.

2. Set Learning Goals

Set specific, measurable goals for your learning and personal development. Whether it's mastering a new skill, learning a new language, or exploring a new hobby, having clear goals gives you direction and motivation to keep moving forward.

3. Seek Out New Experiences

Step out of your comfort zone and challenge yourself to try new things. Whether it's traveling to a new destination, trying a new form of exercise, or learning a new instrument, pushing yourself beyond your limits helps you grow and adapt to new situations.

4. Stay Flexible and Adapt to Change:

Embrace change as a natural part of life and stay flexible and adaptable in the face of uncertainty. Instead of resisting change, see it as an opportunity for growth and transformation, and approach new challenges with curiosity and optimism.

5. **Reflect on Your Learning Journey**

Take time to reflect on your learning journey and celebrate your progress and achievements. Keep a journal or reflective log where you can document your experiences, insights, and lessons learned along the way.

Staying Agile and Flexible in the Face of Change

In the journey of life, change is the only constant. Whether it's in our personal lives, careers, or the world around us, change is inevitable and often unpredictable. In order to thrive in the face of change, we must cultivate a mindset of agility and flexibility, embracing new opportunities, challenges, and experiences with openness and resilience. This chapter explores the importance of staying agile and flexible in the face of change for lifelong learning and adaptability, providing insights and strategies for navigating life's transitions with grace and confidence.

Conclusion

Celebrating Your Journey to Mobility Mastery and Looking Ahead to a Life of Freedom and Vitality

As we come to the culmination of our exploration into the world of mobility mastery, it's a momentous occasion to celebrate the incredible journey we've undertaken together. From the inception of our quest to unlock the secrets of mobility to the profound insights gained through mastering the ten essential habits, our adventure has been one of growth, transformation, and empowerment. Now, as we stand on the precipice of a new beginning, let us take a moment to commemorate our achievements and cast our gaze towards a future filled with freedom, vitality, and limitless possibilities.

Throughout the pages of this book, we have embarked on a journey of self-discovery and empowerment, guided by the principles of mobility mastery. Each chapter has served as a beacon of light, illuminating the path towards greater freedom and vitality and empowering us to unleash our full potential. We have learned how daily movement rituals can invigorate our bodies and minds, how mindful stretching practices can enhance our flexibility and mobility, and how strength training can build a solid foundation for stability and resilience. We have delved into the importance of joint mobility and flexibility, balance, posture alignment, nutrition, recovery, and the mind-body connection, recognizing each as a vital component of our overall well-being.

But beyond the practical techniques and exercises, this book has been about more than just physical mobility. It's been about reclaiming our power, embracing our innate potential, and living life on our own terms. It's been about breaking free from the constraints that hold us back and stepping into a life of boundless freedom and vitality.

The title of this book, ***"Unleash Your Mobility: Mastering the Ten Essential Habits for a Life of Freedom and Vitality,"*** encapsulates the essence of our journey. It's a rallying cry, a declaration of empowerment, and a testament to the transformative power of intentional living. It's about recognizing that we have the power within us to shape our lives according to our deepest desires and aspirations.

As we reflect on our journey, it's important to acknowledge the challenges we've faced along the way. There may have been moments of doubt, setbacks, and obstacles that seemed insurmountable. But through perseverance, determination, and a commitment to growth, we've overcome each challenge and emerged stronger and more resilient than before.

And so, as we celebrate our achievements, let us also look ahead to the future with hope and anticipation. Let us envision a life filled with freedom, vitality, and endless possibilities. Let us imagine ourselves moving through the world with grace and ease, embracing each moment with joy and gratitude.

As we embark on this new chapter of our journey, let us carry with us the lessons we've learned and the habits we've cultivated. Let us continue to prioritize our health and well-being, nurturing our bodies, minds, and spirits with care and intention. Let us stay committed to lifelong learning and growth, embracing change as a natural and inevitable part of the human experience. And let us never forget the power that lies within us to shape our lives according to our deepest desires and aspirations.

In closing, I want to express my deepest gratitude to you, the reader, for joining me on this transformative journey. It has been an honor and a privilege to accompany you on this path towards greater freedom and vitality. May your journey be filled with joy, discovery, and endless possibilities. And may you continue to move freely and live fully, now and always.

Thank you, and congratulations on your journey to mobility mastery and a life of freedom and vitality.